# A Parkinson's Life

## And a Caregiver's Roadmap

**Jolyon E. Hallows**

This publication is a personal memoir which reflects the author's experiences and which may contain information of value. It is provided with the understanding that the author is not a health care or medical professional, nor is he engaged in rendering legal, medical, or any other professional services. Anyone who requires legal advice or other expert assistance should seek the services of a competent professional.

Book title:          A Parkinson's Life
Book subtitle:       And a Caregiver's Roadmap
Author:              Jolyon E. Hallows

Publisher's address and contact information
        WCS Publishing
        4210 Rumble Street
        Burnaby, BC  V5J 1Z8
        Canada
        604-683-0767
        Visit our website at www.AParkinsonsLife.com.


ISBN-13: 978-0-9950259-0-5 (Softcover book)
         978-0-9950259-1-2 (Kindle format e-book)
         978-0-9950259-2-9 (EPUB format e-book)
         978-0-9950259-3-6 (PDF format e-book)




Editing by          Joyce Gram
Book design by       Jim Bisakowski
Cover design by      Julie Kitsulie
Indexing by          Margaret de Boer

First Edition: November 2017
10 9 8 7 6 5 4 3 2 1

*For Sandra,*

*who made this book necessary*

# Contents

PART III

# CAREGIVING

# Prologue: The News

D o you remember where you were when . . .?
      That sentence usually ends with some event that made history: an invasion, an assassination, a natural disaster. But it can also end with a personal event: one that nobody outside your circle of friends or family will ever hear of or care about, but one that wrenches your life onto a track you never even knew existed.

My wife, Sandra, and I were strolling toward a path called Rhododendron Walk in Central Park near our home in Burnaby, British Columbia. She had been quiet, had said little for almost a week, which was unusual for her. I was about to find out why.

She tightened her grip on my hand and said, "I went to see a doctor yesterday. He told me I have Parkinson's disease."

Looking back, I don't recall having any kind of emotional reaction to what she said. I'd heard of Parkinson's, of course. I knew it had something to do with tremors. I'd seen film clips of people who were afflicted with the disease frozen as they tried to cross a room. But her words didn't seem to sink in. Maybe it was because I couldn't reconcile these images of infirmity with this woman who was always one step ahead of me. Maybe it was because I had no idea what this diagnosis meant for her and for our lives. Or maybe it was because I just needed time for information like this to register. Whatever the reason, based on my reaction, she might just as well have announced that her hairdresser said she needed to get a haircut.

Still, I remember exactly where I was when she told me.

# Digression

I haven't written an introduction to this book because I don't like reading them, but it will be helpful for you to understand how I've laid it out.

Part I has six chapters. Each chapter in Part I has two sections. The first section tells about Sandra and me from the time we met to when Sandra was diagnosed with Parkinson's. The second section describes aspects of Parkinson's: what it is, its symptoms, and its treatments.

Part II tells of Sandra's journey from her diagnosis to now. It's roughly chronological.

Part III deals with caregiving and the things I've learned. I hope it's useful to you. The book also has some appendices, one of which is Sandra's chronology. It identifies the chapters in which I describe the events that marked her journey.

Part I

# Prelude

# 1

# First Contact

I first saw Sandra at an outdoor party at the student nurses' residence of the Calgary General Hospital in Calgary, Alberta. She was sitting beside a campfire with several of her classmates, and as if ignoring the laws of optics, the light from the fire shone only on her; her friends were in shadow. She was laughing, her face aglow with life. I would learn that was part of her personality.

I was entranced. The song "Some Enchanted Evening" from *South Pacific* played in my mind. I wanted to "fly to her side" and if not make her my own, then at least get to know her. But I had a problem: I had awakened with a tickle in my throat and a trickle in my nose. That was the best I'd feel all day. By the evening, I had the pallor of a parsnip, and I feared that if I fell down at the hospital, some earnest intern would perform an autopsy on me before I could protest. I should have stayed in bed, but my roommate had insisted we go to the party to meet new women because, as he lamented, we'd both struck out with the ones we knew.

While I longed to approach this woman who had so captivated me, I didn't want her first reaction to me to be "Oh, no. Another patient." So I backed away, got in my car, and drove home. I knew I'd see her again. I knew where she lived.

"Again" came sooner than I'd expected when, a couple of days later, my roommate announced he was bringing his new girlfriend over to the apartment. I wasn't sure why. His hobby was rebuilding the motor of his sports car, and since he didn't have a garage, he was using our living-room floor. As centerpieces go, it was unique, although I doubted it would appeal to a woman who wasn't interested in spark plug gaps or ignition timings. But I didn't care; where he took his dates was none of my business.

Then he walked in with her, and I was slammed with three emotions: delight at seeing her again, envy at my roommate, and frustration at the code that says you don't poach your friends' girls.

I wanted to say something pithy, something memorable, something that would let her know I wasn't just another grunt. I wanted to make an impression, but in the stew of my emotions, spiced by the remnants of my cold, the best I could do was to point to the pedal pushers she was wearing and ask her why she didn't have clothes that fit.

Her scowl told me I had made an impression.

It would be a couple of weeks before I saw her again, this time at a disco where a group of us had agreed to meet, along with some of the student nurses. I found out later that she came only because she'd learned that my roommate, with whom she'd had an emphatic breakup (yes!), was out of town. However, she did ask her friends to keep me away from her.

No way. My cold was gone and my judgment was as good as it ever gets, and this time I wasn't going to miss the chance to get to know her.

I asked her to dance, and while the rest of our friends were jiving and bopping around the floor, we somehow slid into dancing the foxtrot. We got a lot of frowns and snickers, but to me they sprang from envy. I was, after all, the only man in the room holding a woman in his arms.

We discovered that we wanted to talk, but the blare of the disco made that impossible. So we went out into the night, next door to a twenty-four-hour coin laundry where we sat on tacky chairs and made up new uses for plastic garbage bags, none of which I recall except that some of them had to do with small furry animals.

I learned that her name was Doris Sandra Adell Johnson. Yes, that's how she spelled Adell; her father, when he registered her, hadn't known how it was normally spelled. I thought it was charming. When I asked her why she had three given names, she told me she had eight siblings, and she figured her parents thought that if they used up all the available names, they'd stop having kids. It must have worked because she was the second youngest.

She was from rural Saskatchewan. She'd come to Alberta to take the province's dual diploma program in psychiatric and general duty nursing. The general duty part, which would give her the RN certification, was at the Calgary General, but the program was based out of the Alberta psychiatric hospital at Ponoka. When I got home that night, I looked up Ponoka on the roadmap. I had a feeling I'd be spending a lot of time traveling there and back.

## All about Parkinson's Disease

Parkinson's disease is named after the English doctor James Parkinson, not because he had it, but because he described it in his 1817 work, *An Essay on the Shaking Palsy.*[*] Of course, the disease didn't first appear in 1817; it's described in records that go back to antiquity. For Dr. Parkinson, getting his name attached to it was just good timing.

Parkinson's disease, characterized by tremors and stiffness, results when neurons in an area of the brain called the substantia nigra fail to produce enough of the neurotransmitter dopamine.

Now, often when I read sentences like that last one, it means as much to me as if the writer had said something like "tIqjaj yInllj 'ej bIchepjaj." (That's "Live long and prosper" in Klingon.) Since one of my goals in this book is to provide an insight into Parkinson's that may at times be irreverent, occasionally whimsical, but always accurate and clear, I need to decode that sentence.

So here it is again in its basics: Parkinson's disease results when neurons in the substantia nigra fail to produce enough of the neurotransmitter dopamine. Understanding this means understanding how the human brain works. This shouldn't take long.

The human brain is composed of gazillions of brain cells, or neurons, which are connected together into a vast number of massive networks. The networks are themselves interconnected, which makes things even more complicated.

A neuron receives a stimulus, usually from another neuron, and converts it into an electrical impulse that travels along the neuron to its end. There, the stimulus is passed on to other neurons, sometimes up to a thousand of them. A neuron's sole job is to receive a stimulus and pass it along,

---

[*] Parkinson. A note on my footnotes. Where I give a name, such as in this case, the complete reference is in the bibliography, which is in alphabetical order. Sometimes I have referenced the name in a comment. The name could also be that of a website or an organization, which I've also included in the bibliography.

like a member of a bucket brigade, although one that's fighting up to a thousand fires at a time.

But researchers discovered there's a gap between neurons that the signal can't cross. So how does it get to the next neuron? Here's what happens: When the electrical signal reaches the end of the neuron, it triggers the release of a chemical. Like a ferry crossing a river, that chemical crosses the gap to the receiving neuron. There, it triggers a new electrical signal. That new signal travels to the end of its neuron and stimulates the release of its chemical, which crosses over to the next one and so on and so on.

Because these chemicals transmit neurological signals, they're called "neurotransmitters." Researchers have identified about a hundred of them and similar chemical messengers.* One of them is dopamine. A deficiency of dopamine leads to Parkinson's.

Dopamine is one of the so-called "feel good" neurotransmitters; an abundance of it is associated with feelings of euphoria and well-being.† On the other hand, levels that are too high are associated with schizophrenia.‡ So getting the level of dopamine right is a balance between voices in your head and tremors in your hand.

And that's it. Whether your brain is balancing your blood sugar or balancing you, whether you're composing a symphony or planning a genocide, it's all networks of neurons passing along electrical signals.

Okay, you may say, but what about this substantia nigra thing? "Substantia nigra" is Latin for "black substance," an example of how medicine—and law—love Latin words: they sound so much more impressive.

The substantia nigra is a region of the brain that is responsible for, among other things, overseeing motor control and coordination. When it detects that you need some motor control or coordination, it sends out signals from its neurons to those in other areas of the brain. Like memos that a clerk is routing around an office, these signals stimulate other neurons until some of them trigger movements in the muscles that need to be moved. This system is what allows you to stand upright, jump up and down, catch a ball, and drink a cup of coffee without spilling it down your front. When there's not enough dopamine to carry the signals to other areas of the brain,

---

\*     Cherry.

†     There are four others: serotonin, GABA (gamma-Aminobutyric acid), norephinephrine, and acetylcholine.

‡     Birtwhistle.

or even when there's not enough dopamine to transmit the signals within the substantia nigra itself, the system malfunctions and you have a loss of motor control and coordination. You have Parkinson's disease.

So there you have it. Parkinson's disease results when neurons in the substantia nigra fail to produce enough of the neurotransmitter dopamine.

I must note here that many references state that Parkinson's results when the dopamine-producing neurons in the substantia nigra die. I have a couple of problems with that. First, to speak of "dopamine-producing neurons" implies there is a repository of dopamine for other neurons to use. Not true: each neuron produces its own neurotransmitters. Second, if the neurons die, how would giving dopamine medications help? Dead neurons can't use them—giving them would be like tube-feeding a corpse—and live neurons don't need them. These neurons do die, but before they do so, they fail to produce enough dopamine to consistently carry the signals to other parts of the brain.

But there are a couple of nagging problems. One of the symptoms of Parkinson's is an abundance of movements you don't want, such as tremor, while another is an impairment of movements you do want, such as walking. Why? Why do the hands shake but the legs freeze?

Some intriguing speculation* has suggested that perhaps freezing is a logical response of the brain. Different neurons use different neurotransmitters, but only 30,000 to 50,000 use dopamine.† (Neuroscientists refer to these neurons as "dopaminergic." From here on, I'll just call them "dopamine neurons.") With about a hundred billion neurons in the brain, that's the equivalent of 100 to 150 people in the entire United States—and they all live in the same town, probably somewhere in New Mexico. There may not be a lot of these neurons, but they reach to almost all areas of the brain, and in addition to motor control, they form part of the reward system.

Let's say you pass a storefront in the mall and you see something in the window that interests you. Do you go into the store to examine it or do you move on? It all depends. Do you have the money? Is there someone waiting for you at the coffee shop? Are you in a hurry? Do you really need, or want, whatever this is? The evaluation of each alternative—to go into the store or to move on—is one of the things the dopamine neurons provide. They help us choose.

---

*   Montague, pages 156–158.

†   Montague, page 106.

But what happens when the signals fail? In that case, there's nothing to tell the brain what to do. So, lacking direction, it does the logical thing: it waits—it freezes. When Parkinson's damages the dopamine neurons, it damages not only motor control but also the ability to value choices, one of the most important parts of our daily lives. Now, I must point out that this idea is speculative, and in watching Sandra, it doesn't always appear to be apt, but there are times when she struggles to choose between options that would not have given her a second's pause before the disease.

The second nagging problem is this: as researchers dig deeper into Parkinson's, they are finding out that it's far more complicated than a dopamine deficiency, despite the claims of most consumer information and websites. They've discovered that as the disease progresses, it damages not only the substantia nigra but also other areas of the brain, leading one researcher to suggest a novel hypothesis: that Parkinson's has six stages,[*] each one occurring as the disease moves on to affect different parts of the brain. These stages occur in the same sequence for all Parkinson's patients. The substantia nigra isn't affected until stage 3, which implies that Parkinson's begins long before the typical symptoms start to appear.

But not all is sweetness and light in research-land. Some other researchers have said, in effect, "This is a crock."[†] (Their actual words were more genteel. At university, Sandra analyzed a theory she thought was nonsense, but instead of calling it nonsense, she wrote, "One has to question the assumption that . . ." Her professor, who also thought the idea was nonsense, was delighted.)

The researchers who question the idea of six fixed stages don't dispute that various parts of the brain are affected, nor do they question which parts. But since there's no relationship between these stages and the actual symptoms of the disease, they argue it's wrong to suggest it advances so systematically.

So who's right? I don't know. I'm not qualified even to have an opinion. But one thing is clear to me: this argument isn't about the extent to which Parkinson's affects different areas of the brain; it's a debate about how it progresses. So to me and probably to you, it doesn't matter. What does matter is that Parkinson's is far more complex than researchers had suspected and that it will be a long time before there's a cure on the horizon.

---

[*]    Braak.

[†]    Burke.

# 2

# Getting to Know You

The more I got to know Sandra, the more she fascinated me. She was different from other women I'd met because she didn't know the rule or, more likely, chose to ignore it. What rule?

This was the mid-1960s, a time when women were regarded as suitable for menial tasks, but don't let them near anything important. It was a time when it was unusual for a woman to drive a car; unthinkable for her to have a male passenger. It was a time when my boss could say to a roomful of employees that he'd never hire a woman as a computer programmer because women couldn't think logically—and not get contradicted, hooted down, or reported to a human rights commission.

And it was a time when women were taught the rule: never best a man—not in a game, never in a debate. Men, they were taught, wouldn't have anything to do with women who were smarter than they were. So, my dear, if you don't want to endure your dotage knitting booties for other people's grandchildren, always let the fragile male ego win. (I've always felt this attitude demeans men more than women. But then, I'm a man, cursed with a fragile male ego.)

The rule was frustrating. Many times, I'd debate with a woman about some topic, usually one she was more qualified than I was to discuss, and she'd have me, she'd made her point. All she had to do was jump up and down, hoot, and claim victory. But her eyes would glaze over, the rule would rise in her head, and she'd mutter something like, "Well, maybe you're right." Was there a woman who would stand up for herself? Who would ignore the rule?

I realized my search was over the first time I argued about something with Sandra. I think the debate had to do with health care, her specialty, and she'd won. Her logic and knowledge were superior to mine, and she knew how to express them in a way that left me no wriggle room. But just when I expected the rule to kick in, she pounced. Not only had she won, she made it clear she'd been dealing with someone who didn't know what he was talking about. She triumphed, she was proud of it, and she celebrated her victory.

I was fascinated. Chagrined, but fascinated.

Over time, I found out more about her and how she dealt with her world. I learned that she had contempt for authority, particularly when it was ill-informed. She was working at a nursing station when a supervisor stormed up and snapped at her that room 123 was a mess, the bed was untidy, and it was nowhere near the level of quality that the hospital expected. She demanded Sandra go into the room, now, and fix it.

Sandra walked into the room, looked around, thought *Seems fine to me*, and returned to the nursing station without touching anything. Half an hour later, the supervisor reappeared and pronounced that the room was now up to standard and she expected that level of performance in the future. Even as she promised to provide it, Sandra didn't bother to look up from the chart she was working on.

Her judgment was not only excellent, it was instant. While in training at Ponoka, she was the lone staff member on a locked psychiatric ward when one of the patients began to act up. Sandra was able to restrain her, but the other patients were becoming restive and she saw she needed help. She couldn't leave the patient she was restraining, so she tossed her keys to a patient she trusted and told her to get more staff.

Giving the keys to a patient on a locked ward is forbidden, taboo, a firing offense, so she expected to be reprimanded or even kicked out of the program. But she never heard a word from anyone. Nobody congratulated her on her judgment, but not being hauled onto the carpet was evidence to her that her instructors thought she'd made the right choice, not only for her safety but also for that of the patients on the ward.

She was willing to take serious action when it was needed. On a general duty ward, a young boy was terrorizing other patients and the staff. He would pour ice water inside the casts of patients with broken bones, or adjust the flow of intravenous medications, either stopping it or turning it full on. All attempts to get him under control had failed, including talking with his parents, who said he was simply expressing himself and the staff were not to interfere with his social development. Sandra couldn't let this kid put people at risk, so after he endangered yet another patient with one of his stunts, she pulled him aside into a supply room and gave him a light spanking. The boy never acted out again when she was on the ward. When another staff member noticed and asked why, Sandra just smiled and said she had a way with children. (When I've told others this story, some people criticized her for what they called "assault," and they criticized me for approving of it. Sandra was a nurse, and she saw it as her responsibility to ensure the safety and well-being of the patients in her care. Getting this kid to stop was one of those responsibilities. I hope that if I'm ever in hospital, the nurses there have the same attitude.)

Sandra was also quick to respond. I had arranged to meet her for lunch, and I was walking to the restaurant with someone from my office when I saw her coming toward us. I said, "There's a cute chick. I think I'll pick her up." My co-worker looked at me askance as I strode up to her and said, "Hi there, lady. Would you like to have lunch with me? Then we can go back to my place and fool around." She said, "Sure, mister. That sounds like fun." She slipped her arm into mine and we walked into the restaurant. I grinned back at my co-worker, standing on the sidewalk struggling to remember my incredibly effective pickup line.

She had a way with recalcitrant patients. One of them was a pensioner who always resisted taking her medications or would take one but not the other. Sandra told her she had to take them together. When the woman demanded to know why, Sandra said, with a straight face, that the pills were afraid of the dark and needed each other's company. The woman stared at her and then laughed. Never again did she resist taking her medications whenever Sandra gave them.

## Diagnosis and the Search for a Biomarker

What causes Parkinson's? Good question. Parkinson's specialists call the disease "idiopathic." This is not an insult; it's a term meaning that the cause is unknown. I guess using a fancy word is more comfortable for a professional than saying duh.

In small part, it's genetic. Researchers suspected this because Parkinson's tends to recur in some families. They've confirmed their suspicions by identifying some genes that make their owners more susceptible to developing the disease.

However, many people with these genes don't develop Parkinson's and many more without them do. Researchers suspect that toxins play a role, but which toxins and which role and how they affect the brain remain to be discovered. Whatever the cause, Parkinson's affects about one in every 250 people over the age of forty and one in a hundred over sixty-five. Worldwide, there are seven to ten million people with the disease. That's more than the total number of people with multiple sclerosis, muscular dystrophy, and Lou Gehrig's disease (ALS) combined.[*][†]

Related to the question of what causes Parkinson's is the question of strategies to avoid getting it. Unfortunately for modern sensibilities, nicotine and caffeine seem to reduce the risk of the disease.[‡] So go ahead: light up over your daily cup of extra-strength coffee.

Parkinson's doesn't have what doctors call a "biomarker," which makes it difficult and tricky to diagnose. There are no blood tests for the disease, no scans—X-rays, CT scans, MRIs—no electro-whatsis-ograms, no ultrasound tests. While there is some evidence that the disease shows up on PET (positron emission tomography) scans and SPECT (single-photon emission computed tomography) scans, these are expensive, used primarily for research, and not yet available for large-scale diagnosis. So currently, the only way to identify Parkinson's is through its signs and symptoms. (Medicine differentiates between these. A sign of a disease is a manifestation of it that is apparent to a doctor, whereas a symptom is the patient's experience. If you have a broken bone, the sign is the X-ray showing the break, plus, I suppose, your screams. The symptom is the pain you feel. Some, like tremor, can be both.[§])

And what are those symptoms? There are four major ones. The best known and most common is tremor, usually of the hands and often of the legs and head. The second is stiffness or rigidity, in which the patient moves slowly and haltingly, sometimes even freezing, usually in a doorway

---

[*]    Cram, page 13.

[†]    Christensen, page 3. Christensen adds myasthenia gravis to that list.

[‡]    Sharma, page 57. Also Ross.

[§]    Sharma, page 13.

or crowded place. The third symptom is impairment of movements that require the use of fine muscles in activities such as writing or buttoning clothes. The fourth is instability in standing, leading to a shuffling, tentative walk and risk of falling.

Those are the big four symptoms, but there are many others:

- decreased arm swing
- excessive salivation
- feelings of despair or anxiety
- increase in dandruff or oily skin
- lack of facial expression
- less frequent blinking and swallowing
- lowered voice volume
- slight foot drag
- stooped posture
- trouble sleeping
- constipation
- pain
- decreased sense of smell
- muscle aches
- fatigue
- clinical depression
- sexual dysfunction
- obsessive-compulsive behaviors
- visual or auditory hallucinations
- loss of ability to process and understand visual information
- Parkinson's dementia*

Whew. About the only thing missing from this list is spontaneous sex change.

And death. Parkinson's is not fatal; nobody dies from it. They may die from conditions arising from it, such as complications from broken bones

---

* C-Health, "Parkinson's Disease (Shaking Palsy)." This list has been adapted and supplemented from other sources.

when they fall, or pneumonia, caused when food or liquid goes down the wrong pipe and into the lungs. According to one source, this is the most common cause of death among Parkinson's patients.[*] But an otherwise healthy person with Parkinson's can expect to live almost as long as a healthy person without it.[†]

Parkinson's gets worse over time as the neurons in the substantia nigra produce less and less dopamine and die out. It's been estimated that by the time the first symptoms of the disease appear, between 50 and 70 percent of the dopamine neurons are already dead.[‡] This is an illustration of what computer types call "redundancy": how when something fails, there's capacity somewhere else to take over.

In the final stage of the disease, the person is bedridden and needs help in all areas of his or her life including getting dressed, eating, and personal hygiene.

Parkinson's progresses at different rates in different people.[§] In some patients, it appears to take over within a few years, while in others, decades can pass with few symptoms. The main scale for measuring the severity of the disease is the Unified Parkinson's Disease Rating Scale or UPDRS, an acronym that led a friend to say "Up doctors." Whether this was a compliment she didn't say.[¶] The UPDRS consists of up to sixty-five tests, depending on the version. A test might be ease of standing up from a chair, or the degree of resting tremor. Each test gives a value from zero to four. Zero means no problem, while four is maximum impairment. So the UPDRS is like golf: the lower the score, the better. Par is zero.

Another scale used in measuring the severity of the disease is called the Hoehn and Yahr scale. This is far coarser than the UPDRS: it originally had only five levels. Level 1 is no disability, while level 5 is bedridden. The scale has been modified to add two more levels, although for some reason it still only goes to level 5; the new levels are 1.5 and 2.5.

Parkinson's has been called a "boutique" disease, although I prefer to think of it as a buffet because not all Parkinson's patients have the same

---

[*]    Iwasaki.

[†]    Heyn & Stöppler. However, for a contradictory view, see Boyles.

[‡]    Cheng.

[§]    Michael J. Fox Foundation

[¶]    For the UPDRS tests, see Sharma, pages 43–48. Also see Christensen, Appendix 2. However, there are several variants of the test, and it's constantly being updated, so the test you or your loved one takes will probably be somewhat different.

symptoms. For example, about a quarter of Parkinson's patients don't have tremor. Not only that, but every symptom can indicate something other than Parkinson's. Tremor, for example, may arise from multiple sclerosis or from a condition called essential tremor. So it's not enough for a doctor to suspect Parkinson's from the symptoms a patient displays; he or she must also rule out other causes of the same symptoms. After all, if I'm eating chicken wings and you're having meatballs, are we feasting from the same buffet?

One research study[*] found that 15 percent of people diagnosed with Parkinson's did not have it, while 19 percent of those with symptoms who had been diagnosed with something else, did. Another writer reports that the Michael J. Fox Foundation puts the figure of those who have been misdiagnosed with Parkinson's at 20 percent.[†]

The problem of misdiagnosis hit Sandra's family when her oldest sister, Esther, was told she had Parkinson's, a diagnosis that outraged Sandra and another of her sisters, Vivian, also a nurse. One of their objections was that the diagnosis was made by an internist, not a neurologist. For over two years, Esther took Parkinson's medications until the family was finally able to overcome her doctor's offense at having his opinion questioned and get her referred to a Parkinson's center. The specialists there reversed the diagnosis. In fact, their note to the family said, in part, "NOT Parkinson's." The emphasis was in the original note.

So here's some advice if you or a loved one has been diagnosed with Parkinson's. First, don't trust any diagnosis that hasn't been made by a neurologist—a doctor who specializes in conditions of the nervous system, including the brain. Your family doctor may suspect the disease, but only a neurologist is qualified to diagnose it. Having it done by someone else is akin to hiring a sanitation engineer as a chef on the grounds they both deal with organic matter.

Second, get the neurologist's diagnosis confirmed by a Parkinson's specialist or movement disorder specialist. After all, if the diagnosis is wrong— if it isn't Parkinson's—you face a double whammy: you get a treatment that doesn't work, might be expensive, and could actually be harmful; and you don't get treatment for the condition you actually have.

---

[*]    Schrag.

[†]    Christensen, page 9.

This difficulty in diagnosing the disease is one of two reasons researchers are looking for a biomarker. They want to find a test for Parkinson's that any doctor can order and evaluate.

The second reason doctors want to find a biomarker is to help develop new treatments. Of course, scientists want to find a cure, but because the disease is progressive, one of their priorities is finding a way to stop it. After all, if medicine can prevent the disease from getting worse, Parkinson's patients, particularly those who have just been diagnosed, would be able to live a normal life with little or no disability rather than suffer the decline that is their lot now.

But since there's no biomarker, how can researchers know if an experimental treatment is working? There's no way to tell except by giving one group of Parkinson's patients the treatment and another group a placebo and tracking them over several years. The research isn't final until it becomes obvious that one group has progressed at a different rate than the other or there's no difference and the researchers have to conclude there won't be. This prolonged research is expensive—one source cites over a billion dollars and ten to fifteen years to bring a new treatment to market.[*] One study[†] involved 45 research sites, 61 researchers, and 1,741 subjects tracked over six years. The results section of the study reports, "The trial was terminated early for futility . . .." I shudder to think how much this cost. So even if researchers find a real cure, it will take years to prove it.

Which is why it's critical to find something in the body that can stand up, wave a flag, and say, "Here I am. It's me. Parkinson's."[‡]

---

[*]    PHRMA.

[†]    Kieburtz.

[‡]    There is a difference between Parkinson's disease and "parkinsonism." The latter is a set of symptoms similar to Parkinson's except it's not. These conditions aren't idiopathic (having no known cause). Some are side effects of medication, some are induced by drugs or poisons, and some arise from encephalitis. For a good description of them, see Weiner, pages 114–123. One big difference between these other conditions and Parkinson's is that the standard treatments for Parkinson's are not effective for them.

# 3

# Closing the Deal

S andra's dual diploma program and similar nursing training has been phased out over criticism that it exploited students. Yes, Sandra was required to work shifts during her training, and yes, for these shifts she was paid the grand sum of twelve dollars a month, petty change even in the 1960s. The hospital was taking advantage of its students and benefiting from unpaid or low-paid or, if you prefer to be dramatic, slave labor. On the other hand, the program combined theoretical instruction with on-the-job training (she was in charge of wards at the age of eighteen), her room and meals were included, and when she graduated, she qualified for two professional certifications and had no student debt. In contrast, today's nurses need a university degree, receive almost no practical experience, and have to pay off tens of thousands of dollars in student loans on a nursing salary. When the Ponoka program was shut down, Sandra saw it as a retrograde step for the profession.

The people who ran her program were protective of the delicate flowers enrolled in it. All men were suspect. At the Calgary General Hospital, the student nurses' residence was guarded by the Dragon, a middle-aged woman who knew that all men were after Just One Thing. Whenever I approached the armor-plated residence desk, the Dragon would continue whatever she was doing while I stood there feeling like a schoolboy awaiting punishment from the principal. Finally, she would deign to turn toward me and grunt, "Yes?" I'd ask for Sandra Johnson, and she'd insert a plug into a switchboard and announce, "Miss Johnson, there's someone here to see you." "Someone" carried the contempt usually reserved for con artists or child pornographers.

Then one evening, I took Sandra to a formal event. As usual, the Dragon ignored me until she saw me adorned in a tuxedo. She did a double-take. "Yes, sir," she said. "Who would you like me to call?"

I looked around to see who she was talking to, but there was nobody else at the desk, so I said, "Uh, Sandra Johnson, please?"

"Of course, sir," came the reply. She plugged into the switchboard and announced, "Miss Johnson, there's a gentleman here to see you." How about that? One rented tux had promoted me from sex-offender-in-waiting to gentleman. And the aura of the tux persisted. Whenever I approached the desk after that, she would say, "Good evening, sir. I'll call Miss Johnson for you." I thought that one day, I'd shake her up by asking for someone else, but I never had the nerve to try it. I suspected she was armed.

Sandra graduated from the program in September 1967 and moved to Calgary. I'd like to think she did that to be closer to me, but the great job she got would have brought her to the city regardless. She was hired with a few other colleagues to set up a psychiatric ward in the Holy Cross Hospital. To be able to set policies and procedures instead of having to abide by ones in place since the Stone Age was not only appealing, it was a fabulous opportunity.

She moved into a furnished basement suite not far from the hospital, not far from my apartment, and not far from the pub we frequented. One evening when she and her friends were enjoying a drink, some men sent over a fresh round of beer. The women had been about to leave and they had no interest in the men, but they didn't want to waste the beer. So Sandra ran to her apartment, grabbed a pail, and dashed back to the pub. In the meantime, her friends had poured the beer into paper bags and run out the door. They got the beer into the pail just before the bags gave way.

One feature of her apartment disturbed me. She had to share the bathroom with a man in another suite who would take a bath whenever Sandra had washed her underwear and hung it above the tub to dry. She dismissed my concerns, reminding me that handling aberrant behavior was her job. She had a point. Once when I drove to Ponoka, she was in town at a local café with some other people. I agreed to drive them back to the hospital, but on the trip back, she asked me how I felt driving psych patients around. I suppressed my visions of axe murderers and garrotings long enough to get back to the hospital, but I had to admire her aplomb in dealing with people almost everyone else would flee from.

By late 1967, I had been dating her for over two years and I had to confront the big question. My younger brother, Nick, had announced he was getting married just after Christmas to Bev, the love of his life. I told him he couldn't marry before me because I was the older brother. His response had something to do with body parts.

I knew I had to make a decision, but when I asked myself if I wanted to spend the rest of my life with her, my only reaction was that the rest of my life was a long time. How could I know how I wanted to spend it? Then I had an insight: I was asking the wrong question. The right question was whether I wanted to spend the next part of my life without her. I didn't even have to think about that one, so for Christmas, I gift-wrapped an engagement ring and gave it to her. When she opened it, her eyes widened, she looked at me, and she said, "Does this mean . . .?" I answered something like, "Well, if you want to."

It was not the most romantic proposal ever made, but her ardent response left little doubt as to her answer, and on August 2, 1968, we became husband and wife. I believe my vows included the "sickness and health" clause. I couldn't have known how relevant it would become.

## The Parkinson's Pharmacy

Treating Parkinson's ought to be straightforward. Since it arises from a lack of dopamine, it's a deficiency disease, and the standard treatment for those is to give whatever is deficient. Scurvy, for example is caused by a lack of vitamin C. So if you have scurvy, eat an orange.*

Probably the best-known deficiency disease is diabetes, caused by a lack of insulin. The treatment is to take some. Yes, it's more complicated than that, but for most people, taking insulin is the best way to combat the disease.

So the treatment for Parkinson's should be, "Take two dopamine pills and call me in the morning." Of course it's not that simple. How would the dopamine get into the brain? You might think the same way any medication

---

* Irrelevant historical note: Scurvy was prominent among mariners throughout history, no doubt because ships' cooks weren't experts in nutritional science (probably because it hadn't been invented yet). After the link with vitamin C was discovered in the mid-18th century, the Royal Navy began adding lime juice to its sailors' daily rations of rum, thus ending scurvy in the Royal Navy and explaining why we call the English "limeys."

gets to its target: through the bloodstream. You're partly right. The blood-stream will get the dopamine to the brain, but not into it.

The brain is persnickety. It doesn't tolerate some of the stuff the blood-stream carries, so it's protected by something called the "blood-brain bar-rier," which acts like a security guard at an exclusive gated community keeping out the riffraff. Among the many substances that can't cross the barrier is dopamine. You can take all of it you like, but none of it reaches your neurons.

So the search was on to find another substance that could cross the barrier and would act like dopamine or even be converted into it. Enter levodopa.

No, levodopa is not curt advice given to someone married to a dull-ard—I'll pause here to let that sink in. It's a substance that, when acted upon by an enzyme, is converted to dopamine. (An enzyme is a substance that acts on other substances to convert them into something else, much like garlic butter turns snails into a dish that's almost edible.) And yes, levodopa crosses the blood-brain barrier. We can deliver levodopa into the brain and let the enzyme convert it into all the dopamine we need. So the treatment is, "Take two levodopa pills and call me in the morning."

Well, no.

The enzyme that converts levodopa to dopamine is present not only in the brain but also throughout the body. This has two consequences. The first is that by the time the levodopa reaches the brain, most of it has already been converted to dopamine and there's not much left. We could solve this problem by upping the dose. "Take four levodopa pills . . ." but that runs into the second problem: although the brain thrives on dopa-mine, the rest of the body is not so crazy about it. The increased dopamine levels in the body can cause nausea and vomiting, sometimes so severe as to be dangerous.

What we need is something that will stop the enzyme from acting on the levodopa until it gets to the brain. Cue carbidopa. Like a police escort obstructing the paparazzi, carbidopa blocks the enzyme and keeps it away from the levodopa. Best of all, carbidopa can't cross the blood-brain bar-rier. So once it has escorted its cargo to the brain, it stays behind in the bloodstream, no doubt looking for more of the enzyme to frustrate.

Today, the gold standard in Parkinson's medication is levodopa/carbidopa. For convenience, it's usually referred to as "levodopa" or sometimes "L-dopa." From here on, I'll call it levodopa.

There are several brand-name versions, the best known of which is Sinemet, manufactured by Merck. The name "Sinemet" comes from the Greek "sine" (without) and "emesis" (vomiting).[*] It also gave rise to one of the few jokes I have created. The last line is to be belted out to the tune of Elvis Presley's "Heartbreak Hotel."

Here it is.

> Knock, knock.
> Who's there?
> Sinemet.
> Sinemet who?
> Well Sinemet ya baby.

Oh, well, they loved it at the clinic.

Unfortunately, most medications have side effects, results you don't want—although some of them, like reduced blood pressure, can be useful if you need them. But most of them are bad. One of the main side effects of levodopa is called "dyskinesia," a writhing, twisting motion, usually of the head, shoulders, and arms. These aren't symptoms of Parkinson's, but people often mistake them as such, including the well-known U.S. radio talk show host Rush Limbaugh.[†]

During a senatorial election, the actor Michael J. Fox, who has Parkinson's, made a television advertisement supporting a political candidate. Limbaugh, who opposed this candidate, claimed on air that Fox had gone off his medications to garner sympathy. But Fox's movements were dyskinesias: those of someone very much on his medications and displaying the side effects.

Over time, as the levels of dopamine in the brain diminish even further, the medications become less effective and wear off faster, leading to what's called the "on/off" phenomenon. Patients who are "on" have fewer or less-severe symptoms than when they're "off." But as the disease progresses, the "on" times become shorter, and sadly, the "off" times lengthen.

---

[*]  Parashos, page 99.

[†]  Montgomery. For a fuller description of this incident, see Fox (2009), pages 128–150.

There are other medications that can extend the effect of levodopa, but these have their own limits.

A major group of Parkinson's medications is the dopamine agonists. Despite the painful name, an agonist is a substance that mimics something else, so the dopamine agonists act like dopamine in the brain. These are useful, but not as effective as levodopa, and one of their side effects is to reduce inhibitions. People taking them have reported engaging in compulsive behaviors such as gambling, drinking, and sex. I wonder why they're not street drugs.

I've included a list of medications that have proven useful in treating Parkinson's. You'll find it in Appendix B: Parkinson's Medications.

Medications have given generations of Parkinson's patients extended time and a better quality of life, but there's only so much they can do in the face of the disease's inexorable progress.

# 4

# Passports and Other Trivia

About a year after we were married, my boss told me I was too expensive for him. The work I was doing could be done by someone with less experience, less seniority, and most important for his budget, lower pay. So he wanted me to transfer to the company's software development lab in Toronto.

Sandra and I had planned on traveling to Europe and staying for at least a year, and since I'd figured out that Toronto was closer to Europe than Calgary was, we agreed to the move.

One of our priorities was to get our passports. For that, Sandra needed her birth certificate. She got the application form from the Saskatchewan Division of Vital Statistics and was filling it in when she said, "They want to know my birthplace. I don't know what to put down."

I replied something like, "This is just a wild guess, but how about where you were born?"

She said, "I was born in Grandma's house."

"Why were you born in Grandma's house?"

"A blizzard had closed the road and we couldn't get to the doctor."

"Gee, that's too bad."

"Not really. When I grew up, I met the doctor."

I suggested she put down the name of the nearest town, the village of Beatty. She completed the application, attached five dollars, and sent it in.

She heard nothing back. No birth certificate, no acknowledgement, and no refund of the five dollars. So she got another application and filled in her birthplace as Kinistino, the town where she went to high school. Still nothing. So she tried a third time, giving her birthplace as Melfort, the nearest city and the site of the hospital. Again, no response.

At this point, not only were we getting tired of financing the Saskatchewan government, we were running out of time to apply for her passport and we'd used up all the potential birthplaces. Then I remembered that during my early university days, I had wanted to join some friends at the pub. Because I was underage, I did the only responsible thing I could: I asked someone if I could borrow his ID. He agreed and handed over his birth certificate, but his birthplace was a confusing mess of letters and numbers I couldn't remember when I was sober, much less after a couple of beers.

He explained to me that his birthplace was a set of LSD coordinates. "LSD" stands for Legal Sub-Division: a coordinate system for the southern areas of all of the Prairie provinces including Saskatchewan. It identifies a plot of land down to the nearest section or square mile. LSD has no relationship to the hallucinogen, unless, as I suspect, the person who designed the system was on it at the time.

I got some large-scale maps of the area around her home and had her trace the route from Beatty to Grandma's house. She did so, pointing out her place, her uncle Gottfried's, and her aunt Nanny's, until she arrived at Grandma's. I read off the coordinates, she wrote them down on the application, and a couple of weeks later, she received a birth certificate stating her birthplace as Sec.28,Tp.46,Rge.20,W.2, Saskatchewan. Translation: Section 28, Township 46, Range 20, West of the Second Meridian. Higher level translation: Grandma's house. The Canadian government isn't quite so picky. On her passport, her place of birth is Melfort.

When Sandra's parents married, three brothers and a sister married three sisters and a brother, and both families were named "Johnson." All four couples were prolific; it seemed to me everyone in the province was a relative. It made for confusion at family reunions in which Sandra would introduce me to her sets of second double-cousins. I told her she didn't have a family tree; it was more like underbrush. Her family was originally from Sweden, although the only Swedish she knew was the occasional curse and the Swedish words to "You are my sunshine."

She had five brothers and three sisters. All the women but Esther became nurses, which Sandra thought came from having to look after five guys: they might as well get paid for what they'd learned in childhood.

Her mother, Betty Johnson, had been born in Minnesota and moved to Saskatchewan as a young woman. Her father, Sigfred Johnson, had been born in Sweden and as a teenager traveled to Canada where much of the family had settled. In typical teenager fashion he missed the boat and had to catch a later one. It was fortunate: the boat he missed was the Titanic.

## It Really Is Brain Surgery

Aside from medications, there are also surgical treatments for Parkinson's. The most common one now is deep brain stimulation. I'll get to that later. When Sandra was diagnosed, there were two: pallidotomy and thalamotomy. All you need to know to conclude that these are serious operations is that they take place in the brain and that "-otomy" in medicine means "cut." The prefixes name the target region. "Pallid-" refers to the globus pallidus (Latin for "pale globe"—see what I mean about Latin being more impressive), and "thalam-" refers to the thalamus (which comes from Greek instead of Latin and means "inner chamber"). In either pallidotomy or thalamotomy, some part in one of those areas of the brain is going to be destroyed.

You may ask how anyone would come to think destroying brain cells in those spots would help. Doctors had noted that occasionally the tremors of a few Parkinson's patients stopped after they had mild strokes. When the patients died, autopsies showed the strokes had damaged these parts of the brain.[*]

In the surgery, a neurosurgeon drills a hole in the patient's skull, then inserts a probe into the brain to the target. Once there, the probe is heated or liquid nitrogen is passed down it. The effect of either one is to ablate the area around it. "Ablate" in medicine means remove, although the brain cells aren't removed; they're destroyed and left there. But I guess when you're talking to apprehensive patients, "ablate" is gentler than "kill." (They're also not cut, as the suffix "otomy" would imply.)

How does the neurosurgeon know the probe has reached the right spot to ablate? Before the surgery, images of the brain are taken. These tell the neurosurgeon where to insert the probes and how far in to go. But one of the main methods is having the patient tell the surgeon the probe has arrived. Not directly, of course, but when the patient's tremors stop, the surgeon can

---

[*]    Parashos, pages 130–131.

be confident the probe is in the right place. This means the patient has to be awake during the surgery. Since the nerve cells in the brain aren't sensory cells—nerve cells that can create the sensation of pain—it doesn't hurt, but being conscious as someone drills a hole into your skull and sticks a wire into your brain takes a certain amount of courage. Or desperation.

These surgical procedures can be unilateral—one side of the brain—or bilateral—both sides. The brain is symmetrical: the left and right sides contain the same structures. So there is a thalamus, a globus pallidus, and a substantia nigra on each side. Each half of the brain controls the opposite side of the body, so if a person's tremor is the right hand, the surgery is performed on the left thalamus or globus pallidus. If the tremor is severe in both hands, the surgery is performed on both sides of the brain.

Thalamotomy proved useful for controlling tremors, but not so much for the other Parkinson's symptoms. Pallidotomy was used not only for tremors but also for stiffness, where it had some success. It was also sometimes used to lessen the effects of dyskinesias caused by levodopa. However, deep brain stimulation surgery has largely replaced both of these.

The main problem with these procedures is they're not reversible. If they don't do the job or if something better comes along, too bad. But for some patients, having surgery is better than doing nothing.

## Deep Brain Stimulation Surgery*

Deep brain stimulation (DBS) surgery targets approximately the same areas of the brain as thalamotomy and pallidotomy, but the procedure doesn't kill neurons. Incidentally, calling it "DBS surgery" is correct, unlike referring to "an ATM machine." The "M" in ATM stands for machine, so "ATM machine" means "automated teller machine machine." However, the "S" in "DBS" doesn't stand for "surgery"; it stands for "stimulation." So it's correct to say "DBS surgery."

DBS surgery was popularized by a French neurosurgeon who, while doing a thalamotomy, stimulated the target site with an electrical current of different frequencies and noted that the patient's tremors stopped. The U.S. Federal Drug Administration approved the procedure in 1997. It is now being used not only for Parkinson's but for a variety of other neurological conditions. There is some belief the procedure was recently invented,

---

\* For an overview of DBS surgery, see Tuchman.

but citations going back to 1947 indicate that it had been used experimentally for about forty years before it became standardized.[*]

In DBS surgery, a neurosurgeon inserts electrodes into targets in the brain and connects them to a battery called a pulse generator, which can be implanted anywhere in the body, although it's usually placed on one side of the patient's upper chest. The pulse generator sends electrical signals to the electrodes, creating an effect similar to destroying the neurons, except that they don't. The pulse generator is like a cardiac pacemaker, so much so that it has been called a pacemaker for the brain.

There are two big advantages of DBS surgery over thalamotomy or pallidotomy. One is that the stimulation from the electrical signal can be modified. For those of you who are familiar with electrical currents, you'll understand me when I say the frequency, pulse width, and amplitude of the signal can all be adjusted. If not, don't worry. This just means the electrical signal can be altered. Being able to change the stimulus is invaluable because the symptoms of Parkinson's change from hour to hour, allowing patients to modify the stimulus on the spot to fit their immediate needs.

The other big advantage is that the treatment is reversible. The electrodes can be removed at any time, leaving no lasting damage to the brain.

The procedure has become, if not routine, at least standard. Dr. Chris Honey, Sandra's neurosurgeon, wrote in an article, "The various operations of deep brain stimulation (DBS) for Parkinson's disease (PD) are not particularly difficult."[†] If I must have surgery, that's the kind I want and that's the attitude I like in a doctor. I don't want my disease to be the subject of a journal article, especially one that includes the phrase, "Upon autopsy, it was determined . . ."

Let's take a look at the procedure. Different surgical centers have variations on how they do it, but this describes how Sandra's was done.

After she was admitted to the hospital, the front part of her head was shaved—to her, one of the more objectionable parts of the procedure—and a frame that looks like a scaffolding was attached to her head with pressure screws. I told her I was going to take a picture of her that we could use in our Christmas cards. Fortunately for me and my cellphone camera, she was lying down and couldn't get up.

---

[*]    Hariz.

[†]    Honey & Ranjan.

The surgical team then took an MRI of her head to locate where the targets were in Sandra's brain and to set guides on the frame that were aimed at the right spots. The team then took her to the operating room, where the neurosurgeon drilled two holes in her head about fourteen millimeters (just over half an inch) in diameter. Because she was having bilateral surgery, they drilled two holes, called "burr holes," about where her horns would be if she were the devil. (Don't be rude!)

During the operation, she was awake and the frame attached to her head was bolted to the operating table. They then inserted the electrodes. This is a delicate procedure; it is brain surgery, after all. One of the biggest risks is that an electrode will puncture a blood vessel. A burst blood vessel is one of the causes of stroke. The results can range from mild, treatable symptoms to death.

The surgery takes several hours, so one of the members of the team provided stimulation to her legs and arms for her comfort while another monitored to see if she needed mild sedation.

How does the surgeon know when the electrode has reached its target? There are three tests. The first is the depth the electrode has to travel as measured by the MRI. The second, as in thalamotomy or pallidotomy, is the cessation of the patient's tremors. The third is what I call "eavesdropping," although neurosurgeons call it "microelectrode recording" or MER. MER uses a device, built into the electrode, that picks up the brain's electrical activity, displays it on a screen, and plays it aloud so the surgical team can hear it. Different regions of the brain look and sound different, so an experienced surgeon can tell, by the display and the nature of the sound, when the probe has reached the right spot.

Once the electrodes were in place, they sedated Sandra and tunneled wires from the electrodes under the skin of her head and down one side of her neck to her chest. Then they implanted the pulse generator, stitched her up, and went home for a well-deserved break. The operation took nine hours. And it worked. I'll have more to say about the surgery and the processes to start up and program the stimulator in Part II.

# 5

# Our European Sojourn

In December 1970, after about a year in Toronto, we packed our suitcases, and along with our skiing gear and my guitar, we caught the train from Toronto to New York City. From there, Icelandic Airlines took us to Luxembourg (we were supposed to stop at Reykjavik but there was ice on the runway; what a surprise!) and we rode a bus from there to Paris. The next day, we picked up our brand-new Citroën station wagon from the factory. At last, we had someplace to put our pile of things.

From Paris, we drove to Calais, took the ferry to Dover, maneuvered along a set of streets in London with the misleading name of "South Circular Road," and ended up at my aunt and uncle's home in Richmond. There, with the English branch of my family, we celebrated Christmas and New Year's, and in January 1971, we packed the Citroën with camping gear and headed back to Europe for a one-year tour of the continent.

We were relying on a book entitled *Europe on Ten Dollars a Day*. The book was originally titled *Europe on Five Dollars a Day*, but it had been upgraded as prices increased. Today, the low-cost benchmark seems to be a hundred dollars a day. Things worked out well except for the days we actually had to spend some money. When we needed to gas up the car, buy film and butane, and pay for several days at a campground, ten dollars didn't go very far. Around March, after a warm winter in southern Spain, we realized that the only way our savings would last another nine months was for one of us to give up eating. Since Sandra refused to do so, we caught a ferry to England and drove back to London, where I was able to get a job. Since I'd been born in England, I didn't need a work permit, and Sandra, as my wife, could sponge off what the English called my "patrial status."

We expected she'd get a job nursing, but we soon found out that before she could nurse, she had to take a series of courses that would last until our firstborn was in high school and even then would pay no more than what she could make as an office temp. She signed on as an office temp.

Her attitude, particularly toward stuffy office procedures, brought a mixed reaction. On one of her jobs, she was shown a crate, about three feet on a side, into which a mound of file folders had been tossed where they sat in a dust-covered jumble. Her job was to file them onto shelves. She was almost finished when a man in a business suit walked past, dropped another folder in the crate, and started to leave. She called out to him, and when he turned to look at her, she said, "Do you realize that if you put that," pointing to the file folder he'd just dropped, "there," pointing to the filing shelves, "instead of there," pointing to the crate, "then you wouldn't have to hire someone like me," pointing at herself, "to file them, and they'd be available whenever you needed them." He just turned and walked away, probably thinking to himself, "Lippy Yanks." One of the advantages of being Canadian is when we offend someone overseas, we can pin the blame on our southern neighbors. What are friends for?

At another job, she was hired to fill in for a dispatcher at a rubber company, allocating shipments of rubber to customers. One company had been waiting six months for its order, but the production run for that type of rubber was rare, so when she learned that a run was being set up, she called the customer and let him know it was being produced and he'd have it soon.

When she got to the office on the day after the run, she discovered that the managing director had sent the rubber to a different company. She stormed into his office, told him this other customer had been waiting for six months, and how dare he give her rubber—her rubber—to someone else. He stared at her, then offered her a full-time job.

But it was March. We'd been there for a year and it was time to get back to touring. We arranged to have the car shipped from Antwerp to Toronto in June. Then we packed up and crossed back to the continent and to countries where we could finally drive on the proper side of the road.

After six weeks, we'd been to Belgium, Germany, Austria, Hungary, Yugoslavia, Greece, Italy, and Switzerland. And we'd had it. We were snapping at each other, and the thought of another six weeks was depressing. This was supposed to be the vacation, the experience, of a lifetime. What had gone wrong? We talked it over in a café in Zurich. Perhaps it was the pace and we needed to slow down. Maybe it was having to adjust to a different currency, language, and customs every few days. We talked about going someplace like the French Riviera and just lying on the beach. But for six weeks? That sounded even worse.

Then Sandra said, "The problem is that we don't have a purpose. A vacation has to be a vacation from something." I accused her of stealing that line from a fortune cookie, but she was right. We needed a purpose.

Then we recalled we had talked about spending two or three weeks in Paris at the Alliance Française studying French. That seemed to be as good a purpose as any, so we piled into the Citroën, headed for Paris, set up camp in the Bois de Boulogne, registered at the Alliance Française, and became students in Paris. We'd go to class in the morning. At noon, we'd head to the Luxembourg Gardens where we'd have a baguette, cheese or sausage, and wine. Then we'd spend the afternoons enjoying the attractions of Paris, which our student cards made half-price or free. It was a tough life, but we were up to the challenge.

Five weeks later, we decided to add one more country to our list, so we packed up and drove to Amsterdam. After a few days in the Netherlands, we headed to Antwerp where we dropped the Citroën at the shipping company and wished it bon voyage.

A couple of weeks later, we were back in Toronto with my English cousin, Alison, who had decided it was her turn to tour the world. We picked up the Citroën and drove across the country to Vancouver where we'd decided to settle. Not only was my family close by, but Sandra liked it there and it had a definite climatic advantage: in the winter, a blizzard meant a snowfall of not quite an inch, and a cold snap sent temperatures plunging all the way down to freezing. Cars in the rest of the country had block heaters. The garage in Vancouver didn't know what I was talking about.

We decided it was time to start a family. But despite many enthusiastic attempts, nothing happened. We went to a fertility clinic, but this was in the early 1970s when the best they could offer was a thermometer that was supposed to tell when the best time was to, ahem, procreate. We were about ten years too soon, just too early to be able to take advantage of the emerging science of reproductive technology. We talked about adopting, but neither of us was keen enough to follow up.

So we remained childless. It's too bad. After all, Sandra had a way with children.

## Implants, Stem Cells, and Other Controversies

Besides medications and surgery, there are three other areas in which research into Parkinson's is being carried out: fetal tissue implants, stem cells, and gene therapy.

The first two of these are attempts to replace the dopamine neurons in the substantia nigra, and there are issues with both of them.

A problem with any implant is getting it to stay. Like the redneck who says, "We don't cotton to strangers 'round here," the body isn't tolerant of outsiders and will try to reject any foreign tissue that gets moved in, such as lungs or kidneys. The same thing is true of neurons. So however the new neurons are delivered, researchers have to find a way to make sure they are tolerated, like those new neighbors and their taste in what they call music.

The second problem is getting them to work. We may be able to take some dopamine neurons and stick them into the brain, and we may be able to avoid having them rejected. But like recalcitrant kids, they still have to fall in line and do what they're supposed to do before they actually relieve the symptoms of Parkinson's.

The third problem is controlling the new neurons so they don't over-work or become too numerous, producing too much dopamine. That can result in severe dyskinesias. Even worse, dyskinesias that don't respond to medication.

Let's take a closer look at each of these three techniques.

In fetal tissue implant surgery, tissue from fetuses is implanted into the brains of Parkinson's patients in the hope the new tissue will graft and take over the functions of the dopamine neurons. The good news is that happened. The bad news is two-fold. First, it wasn't effective in patients over sixty, which covers most people with Parkinson's. Second, several of the patients, including some for which the treatment worked, developed severe dyskinesias that couldn't be treated by medication.* There is also a big ethical problem: the tissue can only be taken from aborted fetuses, which, for many people, makes this not at all acceptable.

---

* Greene & Fahn, pages 114–123. Also Goldman & Horowitz, page 18.

Stem cell research is a major focus, but to say it's controversial is akin to suggesting that water is damp. Before I wade into the arguments, let's look at why researchers are even interested in stem cells.

Our bodies are made up of different types of cells, such as blood cells, bone cells, skin cells, kidney cells, and so on. Even more complicated, it's misleading to speak of, say, blood cells, because there are three different kinds: white, red, and platelets. And even that's not enough, because there are six different kinds of white blood cells. According to one source, there are about two hundred different types of cells in the body.*

Yet all of us start out with just one. Shortly after "Yes, yes," a sperm unites with an ovum, creating a single cell. How do we get from one type of cell to over two hundred? Because when that first cell divides, it forms stem cells.

Stem cells don't do anything useful in the human body except generate some other type of cell. From these stem cells, all of the cells in our body arise, including our neurons, and including those in the substantia nigra.

So if we can take some stem cells, coax them into becoming dopamine neurons, and insert them into the substantia nigra, we can treat Parkinson's.

The status of stem cell implantation can best be described as "ongoing." There have been no major breakthroughs, but there has been a steady set of encouraging steps.

Consumer alert: several companies on the Internet offer stem cell therapy for various conditions including Parkinson's. Avoid them at least until your neurologist approves them. The marketing of stem cell research allows companies to be devious because there is strong evidence the procedure does work for some conditions, allowing websites to claim success. You can tell when you're being conned when these sites don't tell you the conditions for which their treatments are successful. For more details, see "Evaluations" in this book in the chapter "The Structural Dimension" in Part III – Caregiving.

The controversy about stem cell research arises because the most effective stem cells are those taken from embryos, and some people have ethical objections to destroying embryos for medical purposes. I'm not going to enter this debate here, except to say that when I see Sandra's struggles, I'm not sympathetic to any argument that would deny her treatment.

---

\*    Milo et al.

However, the question is becoming irrelevant as researchers discover other sources of stem cells and techniques to make them more useful. They are even starting to retrieve stem cells from the patient's own body, which would solve the problem of rejection. Curiously, one such source is retinal cells. While embryonic stem cells remain the best choice for research, others are fast catching up.

Stem cell implants create an additional risk: they could lead to uncontrolled cell growth. We call this a tumor. Avoiding tumors is a major target for study.

Recall the three main problems with these areas of research: Will the cells be rejected? Will they work? Will they introduce dyskinesias? If we can ultimately use stem cells taken directly from the patient, the problem of rejection will disappear. As for the other two, stay tuned.

Gene therapy is a different kind of approach. Rather than implanting neurons into the brain, it modifies the genes within the neurons that are already there. There are three areas in which gene therapy shows some promise.* I call these the boss, the teacher, and the farmer.

One objective of gene therapy is to get the struggling neurons to do more: to pick up the slack and produce enough dopamine. This is like the boss who says to his dwindling staff, "We have to work harder—to do more with less. No more wimpy coffee breaks."

The second area of gene therapy is based on the observation that, with Parkinson's, cells in an area of the brain called the "sub-thalamic nucleus" become hyperactive. The sub-thalamic nucleus, or STN, is one of the targets for deep brain stimulation surgery. The hope with gene therapy is that, like a stern teacher slapping down a classroom of miscreants, the STN can be made to settle down.

The third area is an attempt to grow new dopamine neurons, like a farmer cultivating a fresh crop.

Gene therapy actually modifies the DNA within cells; it seeks to replace a cell's existing DNA with DNA that's been changed. How do you get changed DNA into a cell? Well, there is a common entity we've all experienced that does just that. It's called a virus, and the next time you have what I had the first time I saw Sandra by the campfire, you've got one.

With gene therapy, researchers modify viruses so they can't give you whatever disease they normally would, then they insert the new DNA into

---

*    University of California, San Francisco.

them. When they inject you with the virus, it puts the new DNA into some of your cells. At least, that's the concept. Making it work is tricky, and while there have been some successes in other medical conditions, making it work with Parkinson's is still in the future.

# 6

# Life Goes On . . . and Then You're Diagnosed

In Vancouver, Sandra started working as a psychiatric nurse at Riverview Hospital, the British Columbia psychiatric institution, and I hired on with an information technology consulting company. About a year later, my employer offered a temporary assignment in Montreal. We were there for just over a year, but, as in England, Sandra ran into problems getting work as a nurse, partly because of the need to take provincial courses, but mostly because she needed to speak French to nurse in Quebec. While our stint at the Alliance Française had been valuable, she was nowhere near fluent enough, so she decided to go back to school. She registered at Sir George Williams (now Concordia) University to study psychology.

When we returned to Vancouver, she transferred her credits to Antioch University, receiving her bachelor's degree in psychology in September 1978. I told her that with her BA and her RN, she was now Sandra Hallows, BARN, unable to shake her rural roots. She pretended not to be amused.

Several years passed, during which we both worked at various places, including a stint at operating our own software company, when we each decided it was time for a switch in careers. I quit my job and started a one-man consulting company managing systems projects, while Sandra decided to use her degree for private counseling.

One of her passions was hypnosis. She'd gotten interested in it shortly after we were married when one evening we watched a television show about a man who'd had some teeth extracted under hypnosis. There were two remarkable things about this. The first was that the man was a hemophiliac: his blood didn't clot and even a small cut could prove fatal if he couldn't get the bleeding stopped. For him, extracting a tooth had the same consequences as facing a firing squad, only much slower and far more painful.

We might have dismissed the program except for the second remarkable thing: this guy was a friend. He'd been to many parties with us, and I recalled one evening going to a beach and helping him navigate the trail in the dark without falling.

The idea that people could exert control over bodily functions such as blood flow fascinated Sandra, and for the next few years, she dabbled in hypnosis as a hobby. I was skeptical about it until I started to do some teaching and public speaking. The feedback I got was good enough to encourage me to keep going, but many of the participants in the classes gave the same evaluation: I spoke too fast and needed to slow down. (The exception was the courses I taught in New York City. No matter how fast I talked, it wasn't fast enough.) I tried to speak more slowly, but all that happened was that I . . . put . . . more . . . spa . . . ces . . . be . . . tween . . . the . . . sy . . . lla . . . bles. Now people thought I had a speech defect. When I told Sandra, she said she could solve the problem with hypnosis. I'd learned never to reply "Yeah, sure" whenever she proposed something, so I let her do her witchcraft. The results surprised me. The next class I gave, I felt as if there were a governor in my head slowing me down. And it wasn't just a subjective feeling; the evaluations reflected it. They said "too slow," "boring," and "needs to pick it up." I had to go back to her, acknowledge that she was right, and beg her to undo whatever she had done. I could sense triumph in her voice as she put me under.

So in 1994, we opened an office in downtown Vancouver where I would do my consulting and she, her counseling. Because I was out at customer sites most of the time, I wasn't in her way when she had her clients in the office.

She had a peculiar habit I discovered one day when I happened to be downtown. I decided to pop by the office and take her to lunch, but the door was locked. I unlocked it and started to walk in, to be greeted by a scream and a yell to shut the door. She was sitting on the couch dressed only in a bra and panties and eating a sandwich. I said something like, "You must have been expecting me. At least I hope it's me you were expecting." She said that she loved a particular sandwich from a nearby deli, but it was sloppy and this was her way of ensuring that it didn't drip onto her suit. I pointed out that she was risking her underwear and she should remove that too. She didn't follow my suggestion.

Another of her passions was painting. She started when an occupational therapist at the Holy Cross Hospital in Calgary taught a course in oils. The course was meant for the patients, but Sandra and a couple of her co-workers took it out of interest. The result was a painting of a snow-covered mountain above a small lake. We hung it on the wall and got confirmation of how good it was when a friend visited us, looked at the picture, and said, "Hey, Kananaskis Lake is open." The painting is still on our wall.

When we returned from Europe, she took lessons, and I could see the quality of her work improving. When she said she had trouble painting water, I said that didn't surprise me: the water would wash away the paint. She responded by giving me a small but exquisite painting of a wave breaking under a sky that's the same color as the water. It's one of my favorites. Today, her paintings, mainly landscapes and seascapes, adorn our walls.

Then, in October of 1996, she visited a neurologist who diagnosed her with Parkinson's. She was just fifty-one at the time.[*]

## The Echoes of Your Mind

While the physical aspects of Parkinson's are difficult enough for patients and their families to deal with, another set of symptoms is even more devastating: those that affect the mind. There are three main types: depression, anxiety, and dementia.[†]

Many people have said at one time or another, "I'm so depressed." Why? Because their favorite team didn't make the playoffs or someone else got that promotion or someone they care for snubbed them. That's not depression, it's unhappiness. Get over it.

Depression is a clinical condition. People who are depressed may feel there's no point to their lives or that nothing they do will work. Or they may feel nothing at all: a gray void without hope, laughter, or even anger. They may cry a lot or sleep far more than usual or even think about suicide.

---

[*] Younger people with Parkinson's are diagnosed with "young-onset Parkinson's Disease" or YOPD. And what is "young"? Some authorities put it at as early as 40, while others peg it at the average age of diagnosis, or 55. It's arbitrary. For a discussion, see Clarke, page 24.

[†] Davis & Stöppler.

When Sandra worked with depressed patients in psychiatry, one of her goals was to anger them. If she could get them mad, they'd no longer be depressed, at least temporarily.

Depression, like any clinical condition, needs to be diagnosed. Doing it yourself is akin to taking out your own appendix, even if it's less painful.

Just after Sandra was told she had Parkinson's, I started reading up on the disease and learned that depression is a common symptom. I asked her, as my expert on all things medical, if this was an understandable emotional response to having a serious disease or a consequence of impaired brain chemistry. Her only reply was to snap, "It's not going to happen." This wasn't a helpful answer, but I've since found out that even the experts are divided on this question. And she was right. It never did happen to her. She wouldn't let it.

Depression is much like Parkinson's itself. It's hard to diagnose and carries a number of symptoms, not all of which everyone has. According to one source, various studies on the rate of depression in Parkinson's patients have pegged it as anywhere from 7 to 76 percent.* This tells me that even the experts are confused. And I find that depressing. So if you or a loved one is diagnosed with depression, make sure the diagnosis is confirmed by a specialist. The good news is there are treatments for it.

The second cognitive problem with Parkinson's is anxiety. This is also hard to pin down. After all, most of us get anxious from time to time. If the police stop you or your boss orders you into the office, anxiety is normal; a lack of it would be unusual unless you're used to the cops pulling you over or being called onto the carpet.

Anxiety becomes a problem when it has no valid source. If you're anxious about paying the mortgage and you're broke, your anxiety is justified. If you're anxious about paying the mortgage and you have a million dollars in the bank, something else is wrong.

Anxiety can vary in its intensity from generalized apprehension to near panic. You may fret about money when it isn't a problem, or about the well-being of those you love when they're fine, or even about some disaster you can't identify but for which there's no evidence.

At its most extreme, anxiety comes as a panic attack. These are spasms of fear that hit without warning and can cause profuse sweating, difficulty breathing, and a racing heart. Victims of these episodes often believe

---

\* Jha & Brown. See also Veazey.

they're having a heart attack, but the effect is short, usually subsiding after about ten minutes.

One way anxiety manifests itself is agitation. The person becomes distressed, sometimes to the point of crying and acting out, at times throwing his or her arms around in an attempt to take care of the problem, or insisting that somebody do something. Now. What needs to be done isn't always clear because the agitation could be related to hallucinations. This form of anxiety is extreme, although it falls short of a panic attack.

Fortunately, there are also medications for anxiety, so you can intervene if you see your loved one starting to fret about something that doesn't warrant concern.

The third and most serious cognitive problem is dementia. Like the other two, this is a catch-all term that covers a wide range of problems. Unfortunately, dementia has been exploited by moviemakers who use it to create a group of madmen (or madwomen or madthings) to give us all a good scare, especially in 3D. But these portrayals are not of dementia; they are of some form of psychosis such as schizophrenia or bipolar disorder. Real dementia is more prosaic, and sadder.

Dementia has three major symptoms and usually shows itself as a mix of them. One is memory loss, Alzheimer's disease being the most severe. Milder than Alzheimer's but a warning of declines to come are problems with word-finding. We all have times when the word we want is "on the tip of my tongue," and it would be foolish to interpret such brain hiccups as dementia; they're a normal part of life. They become a problem when they're more frequent or when they involve common words that we just don't forget: when we're looking at a dinner plate and don't remember what it's called; when we want to sit down but can't recall the word "chair."

Another symptom of dementia is a loss of what psychologists call "executive functions" of the brain: the ability to plan, to focus, to interpret what's happening in the world, and to make reasonable decisions—and no, you can't conclude from this that someone who makes a bonehead decision has gone mad.

This type of dementia can show up as confusion about time, such as scurrying around getting ready for family members when they're not due to arrive for another week. It can also show up as a leap of attention: when the person you're talking to says things having nothing to do with the topic. You say, "I ran into Fred the other day," and she replies, "Yes, I saw the race on

TV." What's the connection between Fred and the race? Perhaps the word "ran." But maybe not; sometimes there's no apparent connection at all.

Another example is an inability to choose. You might say, "Do you want coffee or tea?" to which she answers yes. Or she might say coffee, but when you deliver it, complain that she wanted hot chocolate.

The third symptom of dementia is hallucinations: seeing things or people that aren't there. Sometimes these can be threatening: some disastrous event is about to happen. At other times, they are benign: someone else, or perhaps even a pet, is in the room. To the person having a hallucination, it's real—as real as anything that's actually out there. There really is a bomb about to destroy the house. There really is someone sitting on the couch. And that person may be an ominous threat or just an unusual visitor. Either way, the hallucination is as real to the hallucinator as you are.

The diagnosis of dementia is difficult because all of these—memory loss, impairment of decision-making, and hallucinations—can range from mild, almost undetectable, to severe. Some people with dementia can function almost normally most of the time; others can't function at all without help.

There are different forms of dementia, usually with different causes. Parkinson's dementia is the type specific to Parkinson's patients. One early indication of it is what's called "mild cognitive impairment," which, as the name implies, is a decline in the person's memory or thinking skills. The decline is slight, not enough to interfere with normal daily activities, but enough to be noticeable.

But I must raise a huge red flag. People of all ages forget things or get confused from time to time, and it would be egregious to interpret a normal mental slip as a sign of dementia. Yet people are quick to do just that. For example, someone misplaces his car keys. Why? Well, if he's thirty, it's a brain hiccup. If he's seventy, it's the onset of Alzheimer's and he'll soon be drooling on the floor. Apparently, seniors aren't entitled to the same mental glitches as their middle-aged children. So if you lose your keys or forget that appointment or overlook that anniversary, don't panic and commit yourself to the nearest psychiatric ward; your medical condition is called "life." Your keys only become a problem when you can find them but you don't remember what they're for.

What makes dementia such a devastating condition is that it changes the person who has it. He or she is no longer the personality, the character, you knew. Over time, it can feel as if you're living with a stranger. And in a psychological sense, you are.

# Part II

# Living with Parkinson's

# 7

# The First Diagnosis

Shortly after we were married, Sandra was carrying a cup of coffee across our living room when her hand began to shake. She steadied the cup with her other hand and set it down on a table. In amazement, I asked her what that was about. She said it was her tremor.

"Tremor? You never told me you had a tremor. I want my money back."

She told me it was an intention tremor that only appeared when she tried to do something that required steadiness and focus. Like carrying a cup of coffee.

I made some comment that it must be hell when she had to give an intravenous—not least for the patient. But she said the tremor happened rarely, and in truth I only saw it three or four times in our marriage.

Then she noticed that the tremor was there when her hand was at rest. So she went to see our doctor, Gidon Frame.

We started seeing Dr. Frame just after we moved into a condo near a mall where he and a partner ran a walk-in clinic. The first time we visited the clinic we saw the partner, and since he seemed to be good, he became the doctor we arranged to see whenever we needed one.

One day when we arrived for an appointment, he wasn't there. I asked Dr. Frame when he expected his partner to show up. The answer was, "He'll be here in seven minutes."

"Seven minutes? That seems pretty precise. How can you be so sure?"

"Because if he's not here in seven minutes, he'll be dead."

*Whoa*, I thought. *I like this guy. Maybe we should have him as our doctor.* The question became academic a short time later when his partner decided he could make more money sticking hair implants into the bald heads of vain rich men and left to start his own clinic. Dr. Frame became our family doctor and has remained so to this day.

So when Sandra's hand began to shake, she made an appointment to see him.

Dr. Frame referred her to a neurologist, Jeff Beckman. Sandra had met Dr. Beckman when she worked at a retirement home in which one of his relatives was a resident. Because her contact with him had been brief, she was certain he wouldn't recognize her. But she did remember him as being a gentle man and one she could trust.

So, on October 3, 1996, she visited Dr. Beckman, who gave her his diagnosis: Parkinson's disease.

Her first response was, "I'm out of here."

She was probably displaying a certain amount of denial: something that's common in any serious disease. For a good description of someone going through it, see Graboys, chapter 2. But despite that reaction, she knew she had to deal with it.

Sandra's diagnosis came as a surprise. Many people with Parkinson's suspect something is wrong long before the diagnosis. Some have difficulties walking or with their arm swing, others report becoming more clumsy, and some experience depression. For them, the diagnosis can be a relief; they finally know what's wrong with them, even if it isn't pleasant. Several Parkinson's patients have written of their struggles with the disease and their suspicions, even before the diagnosis, that something was wrong.[*]

Sandra had none of these conditions, at least as far as I could tell. There was no warning something was wrong. I never saw any need to suggest she see a doctor, and the only indication she had a problem was her tremor that began to appear when her hand was at rest. Her Parkinson's sneaked up on her and pounced instead of sending out scouts in advance.

## The Search for Alternatives

Sandra had one belief I could never accept: she was an advocate of alternative medicine. To me, "alternative" means it hasn't been proven to work; if it has been proven, it's no longer alternative, it's just medicine. But to

---

[*]   See, for example, Levy, Christensen, Fox (both references), and Graboys. (Graboys is a medical doctor suffering from Parkinson's, which gives him a unique insight into the disease.)

her and her naturopath, alternative treatments were viable. She was also spooked by the side effects of Parkinson's medications. Before she would subject herself to them, she would make every effort to handle the disease using natural remedies.

Over the next two years, she would try a cupboard full of treatments. When one of her doctors asked what she was taking, I made this list:

- Vitamin C — 4000–6000 mg/day
- Niasitol (Niacin) — 1000 mg twice a day
- Alpha Lipoic Acid — 100 mg two to three times a day
- Botanical tincture for hypertension (Hawthorne and Dandelion, Ammi Visnaga)
- Acetyl L Carnitine — 1000 mg, once a day
- Ginkgo Biloba — 60 mg, three times a day
- Melatonin — 1 mg, as needed
- Calcium Magnesium — 135 mg, three times a day
- Multivitamins — Three times a day
- Multiminerals — Three times a day
- Flaxseed oil — 2 tbsp. once a day
- Coenzyme Q10 — 100 mg, three times a day
- Vitamin B6 — 100 mg, once a day
- Zinc Citrate — 50 mg, once a day
- Folic Acid — Twice a day
- Vitamin B12 injections 1 mg, twice a week
- Phosphatidylserine — 100 mg, three times a day

I don't even know what most of these are, but she had a rationale for each one based on her research and her naturopath's recommendations. Nobody could ever claim she hadn't tried.

She was able to get a rare appointment with one of the gurus of the alternative medicine establishment. He reviewed the list of products she was taking, congratulated her for the research she had done, and aside from modifying some of the doses, said he had nothing more to add.

But even with alternative remedies, you need to be careful. I've heard many arguments that whether or not alternative medicines work, at least, being natural, they're harmless. Despite being a fan of alternative medicine, Sandra never bought into the "natural is benign" argument. She pointed out that coal tar is natural as is digitalis from the foxglove, and you wouldn't want to eat either of these. Some recent research has highlighted this even more. According to one study, pomegranate juice, which is hailed for its antioxidant powers, actually aggravates what's happening inside the brains of Parkinson's patients.[*]

Despite my skepticism, I had to admit that her logic was impeccable. One study indicated that a substance called Coenzyme Q10 slowed the progression of Parkinson's. When someone told her the findings were preliminary, needing more research, she replied she didn't have the time to wait. If she took it and it turned out not to work, it would only have cost her some money. If she didn't take it and it was proven to work, it would have cost her her health. (It turns out not to be proven to work. In fact, the study to test it was terminated early because of a lack of evidence that it was effective.)[†]

In the meantime, I was feeling like a spectator at an event I knew wasn't going to end well. I began to study the disease, but I couldn't add anything to the research she was doing. I confided to Sandra's sister Vivian that I didn't know what the future held for Sandra and the disease. Vivian, a nurse who had worked in geriatrics, had seen the effects of Parkinson's on some of her patients. Part of me wanted to hear her say it wasn't that serious or it would take decades before the disease became bothersome or the treatments were really effective. I wanted reassurance this was little more than a speed bump in our lives. Vivian's silence told me more about what to expect than I wanted to know. I'm grateful to her for not sugarcoating the condition.

After about two years, I made up a spreadsheet indicating how much we were spending and showed Sandra that, between the trips to the health food store, her visits to the naturopath, and the hits to our bank account for the concoctions he sold her at every visit, it was costing us over $6,000 a year. If all of this had been working, we'd have happily spent that and more, but it was becoming clear to me they weren't. Her symptoms were

---

[*]    Tapias.

[†]    National Institute of Neurological Disorders and Stroke.

worsening, her tremor was strengthening, and she was becoming stiffer and less mobile. She finally reached the point where she had to agree she needed to switch tactics; it was time to accept ordinary medicine. So, in June 1998, Dr. Frame referred her again to Dr. Beckman, who sent her to the University of British Columbia Movement Disorders Centre to have his diagnosis confirmed.

## Clinical Practice vs. Clinical Research

Our experience at the University of B.C. Centre was our first exposure to the difference between clinical practice and clinical research. While this is a generalization, doctors in clinical practice see patients as people with conditions to be treated. Doctors in clinical research see patients as data points to be recorded and analyzed and as subjects for clinical studies. I applaud research and the people who conduct it. Without it, clinical practice would have nothing to practice with. But when you go to a research center expecting to be treated, it can be a shock.

Sandra had an appointment with a doctor who, we were assured, was one of the world's preeminent researchers in Parkinson's, a man with a truckload of citations to his name. Clearly, he was entitled to respect for his talents and gratitude for the attention he was about to bestow on Sandra. He studied her, had her walk up and down hallways, tap her feet, clap her hands, and perform numerous other tests. Then he declared he concurred with the diagnosis. She had Parkinson's. One of us, I don't recall who, started to ask a question.

He said, "I'm not going to answer your questions ask the nurse." Then he left the room. We were stunned. He'd collected his data; we were no longer relevant.

The nurse had peculiarities of her own. The first thing she did when we entered her office was to ask Sandra a question I thought strange, but judging by Sandra's reaction she found offensive. Before I reveal the question, let me set the context.

Sandra ran her own professional counseling service in an office in downtown Vancouver, she ran our consulting company while I was off at client sites, and she had been profiled in *BCBusiness* magazine.[*] In other words, she was a professional businesswoman, wearing a business suit, and

---

[*]   May 1998, page 11.

entitled to the respect she had earned, all of which made the nurse's question bizarre. The question was, "Do you need to go to the bathroom?" In all my years in business, nobody has ever asked me that.

I'm slow to catch implications. Sandra isn't. She explained to me later that the question was a means for the nurse to establish control: we were on her turf. It was similar to wild animals urinating to define their territory. I doubt the nurse urinated around her office, but I did find it interesting that, like a wild animal, she used urination, if only in concept, to assert control.

The nurse explained the options to Sandra, including medications and surgery. She also denounced Sandra's use of naturopathic remedies, dismissing them as ineffective and a waste of money. Sandra replied that since it was her money to waste, it was her decision.

Then the nurse invited Sandra to participate in a Parkinson's clinical trial. She offered two carrots. First, by joining the trial, Sandra would be helping advance the treatment of Parkinson's. Second, the Movement Disorders Centre had thousands of patients—more than the staff could see with any frequency. But people who were part of a clinical trial would get more personal attention and more frequent consultations with the medical staff.

## The Clinical Trial

Let me make a digression about clinical trials and what to expect if you're ever recruited into one.

Clinical trials usually come in three phases called, logically enough, Phase I, Phase II, and Phase III. Sometimes, there are also Phase 0 and Phase IV trials, but the bulk of them are Phases I to III.

Phase I, on a small number of people, a dozen or so, tests to see if the treatment is safe. Phase II, on a similar number, tests to see if it works. Phase III, usually involving hundreds or even thousands of people in hospitals and clinics across the country and around the world, establishes how effective the treatment is and the extent of its side effects. Phase III is usually the last step on the long and expensive route to regulatory approval, allowing the treatment to be offered to the public.

In a Phase III trial, which Sandra's was, the subjects are divided randomly into two groups. The "experimental" group receives the treatment that is being tested. The "control" group receives a placebo: a treatment, like a sugar pill, that has no medical effect. Of course, the hope is the people in the experimental group will do better than those in the control group.

Why have a control group? Why not simply compare the people who are getting the drug to everyone else who has the disease? Because of something called the "placebo effect." The placebo effect is an improvement in a medical condition arising from a treatment with no medical value.[*] In other words, I take a sugar pill and I get better. Of course, I don't know that I'm taking something that's useless; the placebo effect arises when I believe this little pill will cure me. The placebo effect is particularly strong in Parkinson's. One reference reports improvements in motor scores of 20 to 30 percent lasting up to six months just from a placebo.[†] The placebo effect led one writer to propose marketing "placebos": empty pills for whatever ails you. He claims the Federal Drug Administration nixed the idea.[‡]

So if researchers give a new medication to some patients who then get better, did the patients improve because of the medication or because of the placebo effect? Modern studies have addressed this problem by not telling patients which group they are in; all of them benefit equally from the placebo effect. The hope is that those who receive the medication will do even better. This is called a "blind" study because the patients in it are blind to the group they're in.

But even then, there was a risk that a patient's doctor would tell the patient if he or she was receiving a placebo or the medication. This could be inadvertent: a patient who reported feeling better only to have the doctor say something like, "Really? Must be the placebo effect," would know he or she was in the control group and not receiving any real medication. So now, even the doctors and nurses treating a patient don't know what group the patient is in. Only the research manager has the key. This is called a "double-blind" study and is now the standard for medical research.

There's another reason for not telling medical staff which group people are in: the secrecy prevents doctors from pressuring the research team to get their patients into the experimental group so they can receive the hoped-for benefits of the treatment.

People are assigned to one of the two groups by the research manager, and they're assigned at random. Why at random? Because the researchers

---

[*]    WebMD. "What is the Placebo Effect?"

[†]    Fink.

[‡]    Bandler, page 11.

want the people in both groups to be about the same. The same mix of ages, disease severity, smokers and non-smokers, drinkers and non-drinkers, rich and poor, liberal and conservative, gay and straight, tall and short . . . well, you get the idea. By having both groups with the same mix of people, the researchers can be sure the results weren't affected by something other than the treatment. ("Hey, this stuff only worked because everyone in the experimental group was bald.")

So in the clinical trial the UBC Centre offered Sandra, she would not know which group she was in.

The trial was to test a drug called tolcapone, which had just been approved for use alongside levodopa. As Parkinson's disease progresses, patients' "on" times with levodopa become shorter and don't hold until the next dosing. Tolcapone extends the effectiveness of levodopa—the "on" time—so it was being given when levodopa alone was starting to lose its effectiveness.

Normally tolcapone was given only when levodopa became less effective. But some doctors suspected that if they gave tolcapone and levodopa together at the start of treatment, they might be able to give lower levels of medication and the overall effectiveness would last longer. That was what the trial was intended to study. Since Sandra hadn't started levodopa treatments, she was an ideal candidate.

Sandra asked about the side effects of tolcapone and was told they were about the same as for levodopa. So she agreed to participate. She was given a requisition for blood work. To her consternation, it included liver function tests. When we returned to the UBC Centre, Sandra told a nurse she'd done some research on tolcapone and discovered that one of its risks was liver damage. She was unhappy she hadn't been warned about this and wanted more information on just how risky it was. The nurse left the room only to return a few minutes later and inform Sandra that she wasn't qualified to participate in the study. Why? Because she took herbal remedies.

Sandra objected she'd made no secret of her use of herbal treatments, and why was it an issue now and why so suddenly? The response was she was not qualified for the study.

I reminded them they'd insisted herbal treatments had no effect. If that was the case, how would Sandra's taking them affect the research? The response was she was not qualified for the study.

It seemed to us she had been rejected not because of her herbal treatments, but because she wasn't being compliant—a word that had never applied to her. When we left the Centre that day, we dismissed it as having no value for her. It would be several years before we went back. Her disease would be managed by Dr. Beckman, not the UBC Centre.

Because we'd become familiar with tolcapone, we were alert to news about it. A short time later, the drug was withdrawn from the market because of the liver damage it caused. It's since been re-introduced in the U.S. with what the Federal Drug Administration calls a "black-box warning"—a caution that the drug has severe potential side effects.[*] Thanks to the UBC Centre's intransigence, Sandra was never exposed to it.

---

[*]     Watkins, "Tolcapone."

# 8

# The First Decline and the
# First Recovery

In June 1998, Sandra started on Sinemet, albeit reluctantly. ("Reluctant" means dragged kicking and screaming.) She hated the thought of taking it because the side effects of Sinemet include almost all ailments known to mankind. Neither of us had ever taken a potent medication, so we were wary of the warnings and the list of side effects—one website lists sixty-three of them.[*] We've since learned that, probably for liability reasons, drug manufacturers list as a side effect every bad thing anyone taking the drug has ever experienced, even if there's no apparent connection. The authorities encourage this: you can go online to a website of the U.S. Federal Drug Administration and enter a side effect, even if you "suspect" it "might" arise from the medication. If just one person out of the millions who are taking a drug had his left arm fall off, then "left arm separation" will be listed among the side effects. Now I hope this is an exaggeration. I expect the FDA has a set of procedures to evaluate claims of side effects, but I don't know what they are. However, the point remains that some of the listed side effects are rare and may not be related to the medication at all.

Of course, this doesn't mean you should be cavalier about the side effects. When you start a new drug, be aware of the major ones and watch for them. Just don't be concerned that everything on that massive list will happen to you.

---

[*]    C-Health "Drug Factsheets. Sinemet."

None of them happened to Sandra. The Sinemet worked as it was supposed to. She felt better. Her tremors, which by now were noticeable, diminished, and she was more agile than she had been.

Then in 1999, she began to develop severe pains in her wrist. At one point, she was driving and had to pull over because the pain was so bad, so her family doctor sent her to an orthopedic surgeon. Our forearms have two long bones: the ulna and the radius. Normally, the radius is the longer of the two, but in her case, the ulna was longer. This was putting pressure on her wrist, so the surgeon recommended an osteotomy. Remember that "-otomy" means cut. "Osteo" means bone. He wanted to cut a chunk out of her ulna. So in January 2000, just a few days after the Y2K panic was dying out and the hospital was still standing, she went for surgery. She ended up with a titanium pin in her arm and some discomfort in her wrist, but most of the pain was gone.

In the meantime, Sandra continued to work out of our downtown office, doing counseling and eating her lunch in a state of undress. One of her focuses was helping her clients quit smoking. Hypnosis has had good results with this, and most of the clients who visited her reported they were able to butt out.

At this time, one of our favorite events was the Symphony of Fire: an annual international fireworks competition synchronized with music. It had been sponsored by a tobacco company, Benson & Hedges, but in 2000, the Canadian government barred sponsorship of public events by tobacco companies, jeopardizing the festival and forcing it to seek other sponsors. Sandra was outraged and threatened to place an advertisement offering free quit-smoking counseling to anyone who was induced to light up by seeing the company's name on the fireworks barge. She never followed through, but I thought it was a great idea and a perfect tonic to the silly rule that endangered the event and the pleasure that it brought to the hundreds of thousands of people who lined Vancouver's English Bay to watch.

## We Give Up Our Downtown Office

Because our office was near the downtown rail station, Sandra used the rapid transit system to get there. But over time, it was becoming harder for her. She took longer to walk any distance, and it was becoming obvious she could no longer commute safely. So in January 2001, we gave up the office and moved her counseling and my consulting to our home in Burnaby. She still saw clients, most notably for issues such as weight loss and smoking, but her difficulties were becoming more and more apparent.

By late 2002, her symptoms had become severe. Her tremor was uncontrolled, her stiffness acute. I had installed a wireless call bell in the house and was answering her calls several times a day. This did have an upside: I was getting exercise running up and down the stairs from my office in the basement. But she needed help just to get up from a chair, not to mention other parts of her life. Her need for constant care meant I was unable to leave the house for more than about an hour at a time.

She had also developed severe stiffness and pain in her shoulders. She had tried various other medications, including pergolide mesylate, selegiline, amantadine, trihexyphenidyl, and some others that are hard to pronounce, but none of them worked for her. (Appendix B lists Parkinson's-related medications. And I have to emphasize that because a medication didn't work for Sandra, that's not a reason for anyone else to dismiss it. We all respond differently.)

Then she tried a dopamine agonist called Mirapex (pramipexole) and, in keeping with her cautious approach, started out with just a half a tablet. The results were almost instantaneous and almost miraculous. The pain disappeared, and her arms and shoulders immediately became more flexible.

It was at about this time when she asked me to help her with her bra.

"Of course. Always." I said. "But it's morning. Isn't it a little early for that?"

"I mean help me put it on."

"On? I don't know how. That violates my genetic programming. I'll be expelled from the brotherhood of men."

She scowled and said something like, "Suck it up and help me."

I don't know who invented the brassiere, but whoever it was has succeeded in frustrating generations of women who struggle to get it on and generations of men who struggle to get it off.

## The Program at St. Vincent's

One of the most disturbing of her symptoms was rapid weight loss. She had lost over thirty pounds and she looked frail and emaciated. Her doctors did various tests to rule out problems such as cancer. Then her family doctor, Dr. Frame, referred her to a geriatrician, Larry Dian.

In November 2003, Dr. Dian examined her. Then to my fascination, he delivered bad news in one of the most compassionate ways I have ever seen. While she lay on his examining table, he stood beside her, held her hand, and told her she was a train wreck heading for disaster. She was vastly under-medicated. (In his report to Dr. Frame, he described her as being on "a homeopathic dose of Sinemet." Homeopathy is a branch of alternative medicine in which the therapeutic agent—the medication if you like—is present in minuscule amounts, sometimes so low there's not a single molecule of the substance in a dose.) Not only did this fail to quell the tremor, it also prevented her from taking in enough food to sustain her normal requirements. And her requirements weren't normal; the tremor itself burned calories. In effect, she was starving to death.

Dr. Dian also had a recommendation. He suggested she enter an in-patient program at St. Vincent's Hospital to have her medications adjusted to the optimum level. But there was a problem, one that I was sure would cause her to say an emphatic no.

The program was in geriatric psychiatry.

The geriatric part was bad enough. She was only fifty-eight: far too young to be put in that category. But the worst part was psychiatry. She had trained as a psychiatric nurse, and in her career, she had developed skepticism, even contempt, for most of the psychiatrists she had met. She had treated numerous people whom psychiatrists had committed to psychiatric wards, patients who, in her opinion, didn't belong there. She had endless stories of people who'd had psychiatric labels attached to them for the sole offense of being poor or gay or unpleasant or just inconvenient to their families. So I expected her to reject Dr. Dian's recommendation.

But on the way home, when I asked her what she thought and waited for her scathing response, she said, "I don't think I have a lot of choice." So in late November 2003, she was admitted to St. Vincent's under the care of a psychiatrist who also had a special interest in the interactions of medications.

Once we had admitted her to the hospital and completed the paperwork and it was time for me to leave, I asked the admitting doctor where I could pick up my loaner. He looked at me, puzzled. I said, "My loaner. Whenever

I take my car in for servicing, I get a loaner." He stared at me, then burst out laughing. That was a positive sign. Sandra was in good hands.

She was in St. Vincent's for about three weeks, during which I visited her every day and took her for walks in a local park. Throughout the time she was there, the doctor adjusted her medications, the nurses were able to get her to eat, and I could see the improvements almost with each visit. She put on weight, she became more active, and she needed less and less help. After the program was over, I wrote a letter to the hospital with a copy to Dr. Dian. Two paragraphs describe the contrast between before and after.

> Before her admission for Parkinson's disease, she had lost a good deal of weight, she was extremely frail and weak, and she was declining rapidly. She needed help in almost all aspects of her daily life and she was not able to give her business the energy and focus it required. Fortunately, I work at home and was able to look after her, but it was becoming more and more difficult for me to leave home for anything longer than about an hour, and I was facing the prospect of having to give up those occasions in which I had to be at a client's site for even one day. We installed an alarm system in the house with which she could call me from various places when she needed help, and it was rare that the alarm did not sound in any given hour. She was unable to sit upright and repeatedly had to call upon me to help her straighten up.
>
> Today, she is almost completely independent—she has used the alarm perhaps three times since she came home. She needs no help in her daily activities and is participating in housework as well as reviving her business. She is far more robust, and since she has started a physiotherapy exercise program, she is gaining strength. We both know that, until there is a real cure for Parkinson's, she will never be fully healthy, but the contrast between her condition before she was admitted and now is startling.

We will always be grateful.

# 9

# The Cancer Scare

In January 2003, shortly after Sandra left St. Vincent's, she got hit by another problem. A mammogram showed a calcification in her right breast. Was this breast cancer? A biopsy revealed a condition called ductal carcinoma in situ, or DCIS: a pre-cancerous condition that can evolve into the disease if it isn't treated.* So, in June 2003, a surgeon removed a lump about the size of a baseball from her breast. But he wasn't satisfied that he'd removed all of the affected area, so he referred her to the B.C. Cancer Agency.

When we first visited the Agency, the doctor gave Sandra two options: radiation therapy or mastectomy. Sandra said if the condition was only potentially cancerous, why couldn't she just keep an eye on it and have periodic checkups, intervening only if it worsened. The doctor's reaction was instantaneous, as if she'd suggested using leeches. Absolutely not. That was the worst thing she could do. Radiation or mastectomy. Pick one. Or to be perfectly safe, pick both. To help her out of this dilemma, her family doctor referred her to a surgeon who specialized in mastectomies along with breast reconstruction.

Then came what I can only call the sales pitches.

The Cancer Agency wanted her to undergo radiation therapy. According to them, it was benign and no more harmful than a bit of sunburn. Oh, except the radiation would destroy part of one of her lungs and weaken a couple of ribs. The surgeon wanted her to have a mastectomy with breast reconstruction. She even offered to perk up Sandra's other breast as an inducement. When Sandra leaned toward mastectomy, the Cancer Agency told her radiation was preferred for her condition and that surgery had

---

* Breast Cancer.

complications. When she leaned toward radiation, the surgeon gave her a couple of references of women with Parkinson's who'd had mastectomies. We were waiting for either one of them to offer a free set of Ginsu knives—"and that's not all"—before we picked one.

In the meantime, Sandra talked to a couple of friends who had had radiation therapy. Both dismissed the notion it was harmless or benign, and both told her of the effects that continued years later. One of the effects of radiation is to weaken part of the rib cage. This is a serious problem with Parkinson's, where one of the symptoms is an increased risk of falling. As far as her friends were concerned, mastectomy was cleaner and carried far fewer problems.

But Sandra didn't want to have her breast removed. She'd had it for a long time. She asked me what I thought, but the only thing I wanted was for her to be healthy. This decision had to be hers. I know that sounds as if I wimped out, but in reality I didn't like either option, and I would have supported her whatever she chose to do.

She decided on radiation. She notified the Cancer Agency. They made a cradle to hold her in the right position, they marked a tattoo on her chest indicating the target, and they made an appointment for her first bout of radiation.

The day before the treatment, I found her sitting on our patio crying. She said all of her fears were about the effects of radiation and how it would make her life with Parkinson's even harder. She didn't like the idea of mastectomy, but it was cleaner and, other than possible complications of surgery, safer. She had changed her mind. She would have the mastectomy.

She called the Cancer Agency and told them what she had decided, but the doctor, a different one than the one she had originally seen, asked her to come in for one final consultation.

We went in, bracing ourselves for a pressure sales pitch and the Ginsu knives. But the doctor told her there was a third option called "watchful waiting." Because DCIS doesn't always convert to cancer, it was reasonable for her to do nothing. She'd need to consult with an oncologist and have regular mammograms, but in the meantime she could just go home.

When we walked out of the Agency, Sandra said, "What just happened? Isn't that what we originally suggested?" Indeed it was. My cynicism led me to suspect that, having lost her, the doctor at the Cancer Agency was determined the surgeon wouldn't win.

So we consulted with her family doctor, who concurred that watchful waiting was an option, and when we asked for a referral to an oncologist, Sandra insisted on one who didn't do radiation and who didn't do mastectomies. Objectivity, or at least neutrality, was the order of the day.

So in October 2003, she went under the care of an oncologist. His first words to her were, "You don't have cancer." He would treat her until he retired in 2011. She has had regular mammograms and regular consultations since, and she is taking the anti-cancer drug Tamoxifen. She remains cancer free, with both breasts intact and the only sign of her bout with the condition is a small tattoo on her chest where the radiation would have entered her.

Two further points I need to make. First, there is no relation between her Parkinson's and her DCIS. Having one doesn't affect your chances of having the other.

Second, Sandra adopted watchful waiting not because of her Parkinson's but because it made medical sense, having nothing to do with the disease. I emphasize this because I don't want readers to conclude that treating cancer aggressively is a bad idea for Parkinson's patients. If you or a loved one has cancer, treat it.

# 1 0

# Deep Brain Stimulation

In 2002, my mother called and said she'd seen a report on the television news about a treatment for Parkinson's called deep brain stimulation. I looked it up, and on a visit to Sandra's neurologist, Dr. Beckman, I asked him about it. He said it showed promise and there was a neurosurgeon in Vancouver who was doing it. But in his opinion, it was still experimental, and he suggested we wait until it was proven.

Sandra had no interest in anything that involved someone poking around inside her brain, but any treatment that promised to help her seized my interest. I joined an online Yahoo forum for DBS surgery* whose members gave me an abundance of insights into it, including its risks, its benefits, and some principles to help evaluate a surgical center.

A year later, armed with more information about the procedure, we broached the topic again with Dr. Beckman, and this time he referred us to the neurosurgeon Dr. Chris Honey. In that year, I had learned what I could about DBS and had started discussing it with Sandra. What I read convinced me the surgery held promise, but I wasn't the one who needed convincing. So it was time for my sales pitch, which, like some form of water torture, I administered for almost the entire year. It must have worked, or maybe she just wanted to shut me up. Regardless of the reason, she agreed to meet with Dr. Honey.

In our first consultation with him in September 2003, he explained that there were two criteria for the operation: Sandra had to be

---

\*    The forum is called "DBS Surgery." Its website to join is http://groups.yahoo.com/neo/groups/DBSsurgery/info.

"levodopa-responsive," which meant levodopa had to help her; and she had to pass cognitive tests.

To check her responsiveness to levodopa, she went in to the clinic one morning without having taken any of her medications. A neurosurgical fellow—a neurosurgeon training with Dr. Honey to learn DBS surgery—gave her the UPDRS test. Then she took her medications and we went out to a coffee shop. An hour later, after her medications kicked in, we returned and the fellow gave her the same test again. He never told us the results, but I guess she passed because we had a follow-up appointment with Dr. Honey. Apparently, she also passed the cognitive tests.

In my year on the forum, I had been what forum members call a "lurker," an ominous term for someone who reads the interactions but doesn't participate or does so rarely. I didn't have a problem with that since I had nothing to contribute and a lot to learn. I developed a list of questions about the procedure, and on Sandra's final consultation with Dr. Honey, I brought it along. It filled three pages, so I hesitated to ask them, fearing that when he saw the list, he would shut the conversation down. To my gratification, he answered them all, never expressing impatience or an "I don't have time for you" attitude experts sometimes convey. Not all of the answers he gave were the ones I wanted to hear, but enough of them were. (I've included a modified list of questions in Appendix F for those of you who are considering having this done.*)

Sandra had questions of her own. One of them was, "Will I be able to play the piano after surgery?" When Dr. Honey assured her she could, she said, "Great. I've always wanted to play the piano." He still accepted her for surgery.

His willingness to answer our questions and the concern he demonstrated for the welfare of his patients were enough for Sandra and me, and in August 2004, almost eight years after she was diagnosed, she admitted herself to the Vancouver General Hospital.

The surgery carries two main risks: a blood vessel can be punctured and an infection can set in. There was nothing we could do about the first; that was in Dr. Honey's hands. To reduce the likelihood of an infection, we bought new bed linen and we cleaned a set of scarves Sandra rarely used. She would wear them until her hair grew back.

---

\*     For a consensus view of DBS surgery among neuroscientists, see Bronstein.

The stimulator is not turned on immediately after the surgery; we had to wait for eight weeks. DBS surgery often has what's called a "honeymoon period," a time when just having the electrodes in the brain relieves symptoms.

Then, in late September 2004, the surgical incisions having healed, she visited the DBS clinic to have her stimulator turned on. Over the next four months, she visited the clinic several times to have it adjusted.

"Turning the stimulator on" sounds simple, like flipping a light switch. I made Sandra a T-shirt with a light bulb and the inscription, "Batteries included." But setting it is an art with two variables, each of which is critical for how the procedure works.

The first variable is where the electrical current flows. Any current needs two points: one to emit it—the "anode"—and one to receive it—the "cathode." Current flows from an anode to a cathode. Without both, there is no path for the current, and it won't flow.

In DBS surgery, each electrode—the wire embedded in the brain—has four contact points distributed along it. Any one or more of these contact points can be set as the anode and any one or more can be set as the cathode. Furthermore, the case itself, from which the end of the electrode emerges, can also be the anode (although not the cathode). The current, flowing from the anode to the cathode, creates an electromagnetic field, like a puffed-up envelope, that interacts with the neurons it contacts. The shape of the envelope, and therefore the neurons it affects, depends on the contact points between which the current flows. So setting the flow of current—deciding which contact points will be the anode and which the cathode—is the first step.

The second variable is the electrical current itself. Three factors have to be set: the frequency, which is how often an electrical pulse is emitted; the amplitude, which is the voltage of each pulse; and the pulse width, which is how long a pulse lasts.

Putting all of this together is the role of the DBS programmer: someone trained to set the DBS stimulator to the right settings. Out of curiosity, I did a spreadsheet to determine how many unique settings were possible. I came up with over 773 billion, which makes stepping through them a bit of a challenge—at one setting a minute, it would take about one and a half million years to go through them all, by which time the settings probably wouldn't matter. Programming is as much art as it is science.

The programmer will start with a simple setting, then conduct some tests with the patient. Favorite ones include finger tapping, leg tapping, and flipping the hands up and down. The programmer also has to look for unwanted side effects such as tingling in the skin, twitching in the face, or blurred vision.

At the time Sandra had her surgery, the programming at the Vancouver General Hospital was done by neurosurgical fellows. She was fortunate that the fellow present at her surgery was Dr. Rodrigo Mercado, who was from Mexico and would return to the University of Guadalajara when his fellowship was over. Dr. Mercado had the touch of an aficionado: his settings worked for Sandra so well that her flexibility improved and the tremor in her right hand disappeared. Before the surgery, she was taking seven Sinemet tablets a day. After programming, that dropped to four.

At each session, we asked Dr. Mercado to give us a printout of the settings for our records. It's a useful tool in tracking the history of the programming.

Dr. Mercado also programmed her stimulator so we could adjust the voltage of the stimulus. The stimulation acts like a partner to the Sinemet; together they reduce her symptoms. But this works both ways: if the combination becomes too much, she develops dyskinesias. Because Dr. Mercado gave us a range within which we could adjust the stimulus, we could change it depending on how Sandra was doing at the time.

The stimulator came with a remote controller, a device suggestive of a computer mouse. It had six buttons. One turned the stimulator on, one turned it off. The other four buttons were arrows: two pointing down and two pointing up. The arrows increased or decreased the voltage by a tenth of a volt, the up arrows increasing it, the down arrows reducing it. She had electrodes in both sides of her brain, so two of the arrows—one up and one down—were for one side, the other two for the other side. Since the left side of the brain controls the right side of the body, I was never able to remember whether the left arrows were for the left side of the brain or the left side of the body. It didn't matter; we adjusted them in unison.

The controller also had four small lights on the back. Two indicated if the stimulator was on or off, one indicated that the power level in the stimulator was normal, and one indicated when the nine-volt battery in the remote controller itself was low.

Being able to tell if the stimulator is on or off is useful because the world is full of things, such as retail electronic security systems, that can turn it off. So can a magnet, like the ones that most people attach to their refrigerators or like the refrigerator door seal itself.

Security systems and refrigerators seem to have become less of an issue than they once were, probably because there's now an option to turn off the stimulator's sensitivity to magnetic fields so that a magnet or a security alarm won't affect it. But when Sandra first got her implant, having some external device turn it off was a risk, so much so that people with DBS implants were advised not to enter stores that had security gates until the store staff turned them off. I didn't know how this could work. I was pretty sure if I stood outside a store and yelled to the staff inside to turn off the alarm, they'd ignore me. I was surer still that if I was inside the store and asked them to turn it off, they'd call the cops. And I was positive the advice had been written by someone who had never had to live with an implant.

We also had to be careful with airport security. Sandra was given a wallet card exempting her from having to go through the security gates, so when we travel, she gets a manual pat down. I have to say we've never had a problem with airport security staff in accommodating her.

We also discovered an issue with electro-whatsis-ograms. The first time she had an electrocardiogram, the operator studied the printout, frowned, and checked the machine because the results made no sense. We figured out that the stimulator's electrical signals were interfering with the tests. So now, whenever she has any test that involves pasting electrodes onto her, I have to make sure I turn the stimulator off first.

Shortly after the stimulator was turned on and Sandra had a few programming sessions, I showed the stimulator to Sandra's sister Vivian and boasted I could now turn Sandra on and off. She said it was a sorry excuse for a man who needed an electronic device to turn his wife on. She had a point.

Over time, the battery in the stimulator runs out of power and has to be replaced. Sandra's first replacement surgery was in August 2006. Fortunately, this is day surgery and, aside from the inconvenience of not being able to shower for ten days to avoid getting the incision wet, minor. She has since had the stimulator replaced several times without incident. Which is the kind of surgery you want.

# 11

# Speech Therapy and Other Kinds

By 2006, Sandra's voice was becoming soft, so much so it was difficult for me to understand her, especially in a noisy place. I was getting tired of having to say, "I can't hear you. Speak up." Then I found out about Lee Silverman Voice Therapy or LSVT. The therapy was developed by a speech scientist and is named after a Parkinson's patient who had speech problems. It's administered by certified speech pathologists who have taken LSVT training.

I checked the LSVT website,* and in February 2006, Sandra started to receive the treatment from Shelagh Davies.

Shelagh was not only a delightful speech pathologist, she was also a voice coach for singers and for those, like me, who did public speaking and wanted to use their voices to greater effect. One of her interests was working with transgendered people whose voices didn't match their gender identity. Biological men who identified as women still sounded like men and vice versa. Shelagh worked with them to train their voices to match their personas. I have to admit this was not a problem I had ever thought about.

Shelagh explained to us that one of the problems in Parkinson's is that patients lose the ability to monitor the volume of their speech against the background. Most of us will speak more loudly as the ambient noise increases—it isn't just alcohol that causes us to shout when we're in a bar. But Parkinson's patients can't make that adjustment. Combined with the effects of Parkinson's on the vocal folds—what those of us who aren't in the

---

\*    Currently www.lsvtglobal.com

know call the "vocal cords"—their speech becomes soft, sometimes inaudible. The LSVT program focuses on LOUD: getting patients to exercise their voices and to think "loud." Therapists also provide feedback by using a sound level meter to measure how loudly their patients talk.

One of the exercises Shelagh and Sandra did was singing, and for some reason they settled on "Ol' Man River" from the musical *Show Boat*. So it seemed appropriate when, after a vacation in southern Alberta, we gave Shelagh a photo of a bridge over a river. The bridge bore the sign "Oldman River."

Did the therapy work? Yes. Sandra's voice became stronger, and for a time she was able to increase her volume when we were out at a coffee shop or in the mall. However, she ran into a separate problem relating to word-finding.

Because it was getting harder for her to find the right words, her confidence in what she was saying began to slip. As with most of us, when our confidence drops, so does our voice. I told her once that being wrong but loud was better than being right but soft. It didn't work; as her disease progressed, her voice volume continued to drop.

However, one of the tools Shelagh provided was a DVD of LSVT exercises so Sandra could do her voice training at home. While the trend over the years is downward, after each session her voice is a little stronger than it was when she started.

The LSVT Foundation has added a new tool to its arsenal. It now offers physical therapy, administered by physical or occupational therapists, designed to help Parkinson's patients move more smoothly. It has labeled its voice therapy LSVT LOUD and its physical therapy LSVT BIG. Just as the focus in voice therapy is on exaggerated vocal control, so the emphasis in physical therapy is on exaggerated movements.

I found this interesting because whenever I helped Sandra to walk, I constantly encouraged her to take big steps in contrast to the shuffle she would otherwise engage in. "Big steps" became a kind of mantra in our house, and I was gratified when I saw a man helping his wife as he kept repeating "Big steps." LSVT BIG takes this concept and puts some structure around it.

Both LSVT programs are now offered in most cities, either privately through certified practitioners or publicly in hospitals or rehabilitation centers.

# Bones Break

In late 2006, Sandra had a setback. We were walking across a parking lot one evening when she suddenly fell. She didn't trip, nor did she slip. In a typical Parkinson's maneuver, her body kept moving but her feet stopped.

Emergency services took her to hospital where she was diagnosed with a fractured acetabulum. A new word entered my vocabulary.

From the popular song, we all know that "the leg bone's connected to the hip bone." Well, where they're connected is a ball-and-socket joint. The ball is at the head of the leg bone or femur; the socket is the acetabulum. The treatment was to stay off her feet for about three months; she could not bear weight, especially on her left leg.

While she was in hospital, I arranged for a wheelchair and a transfer bench so she could slide into the shower, but my proudest moment was the ramp. Our house has seven steps up to a landing, then one more into the house. I designed and built a wheelchair ramp up to the landing. The ramp had steps spaced one foot apart for traction (this was late fall; winter was coming) and raised edges on either side so the wheelchair wouldn't roll off. There was even room on the staircase to walk up it beside the ramp.

But I still had a problem with the last step. So I built a platform that sat on the landing and was level with the floor of the house. I had installed a raised edge to stop the wheelchair from rolling off the platform, but it was too high for the screen door to open. I considered removing the door—bugs were rare at this time of year—but in the end I put the edge on hinges secured with a hook. It worked wonderfully.

Inside the house, I had another problem. The wheelchair wouldn't fit through the doors to the bedroom, the bathroom, or Sandra's office. Off they came. The only problem was with the bathroom: our guests had to be trusting, desperate, or exhibitionist.

Part of Sandra's recovery was rehabilitation, so we were introduced to Barb Taylor, a patient and capable physiotherapist who came by every few days to lead Sandra through floor exercises to strengthen her muscles. After the rehab sessions, Barb would stay and visit; coffee and chocolate chip cookies were the order of the day.

Fractured hips are often disastrous among the elderly or the handicapped, so I wasn't sure what to expect of Sandra's rehab. Then, on the day Barb deemed her fit to bear weight, we stood her up and helped her to walk. A week later, I was able to return the wheelchair and the transfer bench and disassemble the ramp and the platform. Barb still visited for follow-up rehab sessions, although I suspect it was mainly for the coffee and cookies.

# Seeing Things

Today, it's impossible to detect that Sandra ever had a problem, except for one thing: broken bones hurt. The hospital had prescribed heavy-duty painkillers, which are classed as opioid medications: those that have similar effects to morphine. Sandra was good at telling me when she needed painkillers, and as time passed, she was able to step down to Tylenol 3 (Tylenol with codeine), then to regular Tylenol. However, one of the side effects of the opioids is hallucinations. For Sandra, some of these were severe: an airplane was about to crash into the house or the ship we were on was sinking. I was able to calm most of these fears by taking her to the window and showing her we weren't on a ship or there was no airplane flying around. (Since we can see the approach to the airport from our house, this was a risky strategy.) But even so, at times her anxieties became overwhelming.

I expected that when she stopped taking the opioids, the hallucinations would disappear. The most disastrous ones did, but they were replaced by non-threatening imaginings. She would talk about "her" or "him" and when I asked whom she meant, she would reply something like, "You know, she's right there on the couch." She would hallucinate seeing people or sometimes pets. Her people weren't threatening, they were just present, but seeing imaginary people is something most children give up by the time they reach grade school.

When I mentioned this to one of her doctors, he suggested I play along with her. I have two objections to that advice.

The first objection may seem a little esoteric. Shortly after our marriage, Sandra and I became involved with a group that studied topics in philosophy, and one of the problems we discussed was the nature of reality. (Why not? There's no point in wasting time debating trivia.) Broadly (very) speaking, there are two schools. One is that reality is objective and exists whether or not there are people there to see or hear it. The other is that reality is subjective and depends upon the observer. Sandra and I had no hesitation: the objective side was right. When a tree falls in the forest, there's a tree, a forest, and a crash regardless of who's around to witness it.

We got into a lot of arguments. So much so, that it seemed a betrayal of everything she believed in to pretend people and things that didn't exist were present in the room.

My second objection is more practical. Leaving the house one day, Sandra said, "What about him?" pointing to the couch. Instead of giving my usual response—"There's nobody there; it's one of your hallucinations"—I just said, "He'll be okay." This made her more agitated. No, he wouldn't be okay. We couldn't leave him alone. We had to take him along with us. Now I was in a quandary. I could hardly deny his existence: I had just acknowledged it, but taking along an imaginary friend is a skill I lost years ago.

So now, whenever she comments about someone or something that isn't there, I call it out. I tell her it's just another hallucination. Sometimes she asks, "How do you know?" When I say, "I just do," she seems satisfied. I sometimes wish resolving our other marital arguments had been so smooth.*

---

\*     I have since modified this approach. See the section "Dealing with Dementia" in Chapter 22 in the section on caregiving.

# 12

# Deep Brain Stimulation Revisited

One symptom DBS surgery hadn't been able to stop was the tremor in Sandra's left hand, despite various DBS programmers having tried. We were getting frustrated at some of the programmers: neurosurgeons whose quality of programming wasn't up to the level of Dr. Mercado's. According to the DBS surgery forum, one of the issues in programming is finding qualified and competent people to do it. Many surgical centers have addressed this by training nurses on the grounds that practice makes perfect, giving better outcomes than if it's done by surgical fellows to whom programming is a side issue.

I contacted one of the members of the forum, a nurse who did programming, and asked her if she could look at Sandra's settings. She was in California, but we would have happily made the trip (California in the spring. Why not?). She said she didn't like programming people out of her area because it was difficult to follow up, but she recommended a colleague, Diana Herring, who was a DBS programmer at Northwest Hospital in Seattle.

We consulted with Diana several times. The first time we saw her, she revised all of Sandra's settings, ending with ones that bore no resemblance to those she had had before. To our gratification, Sandra's symptoms improved far beyond what the other programmers had been able to achieve. Then on one visit, Diana noticed that if she activated one of the contacts on one of the electrodes, even with a very low voltage, Sandra's cheek started to twitch. Diana suggested the electrode was slightly out of alignment. Dr. Honey confirmed this with a scan, so in August 2008, four years after the original procedure, he removed the existing electrodes and implanted two more. This time it worked. The tremor in both hands disappeared. Today, she is almost free of tremor; it only shows up when she is under stress.

When the stimulator was ready to be turned on, we learned that the clinic had set up its own programming department with a DBS nurse, Mini Sandhu. After Mini set up the stimulator and completed the programming, we made one last visit to Diana to get her opinion. She left the settings unchanged, and since then, Mini has cheerfully and capably taken care of Sandra's DBS programming.

Although the second implantation of the electrodes was successful, a problem arose from the surgery. Sandra's recovery was slow, and for the first few days in the hospital, she was non-responsive, so much so that Dr. Honey feared the onset of pneumonia. He boosted her levels of Sinemet, almost doubling them to get her to respond. It worked, but her hallucinations slammed back.

I had wheeled her to the ground floor of the hospital, heading for a coffee shop, but she insisted that we go outside. It was a cool day, overcast with showers, but the main entrance had a large overhang, so there was no fear of her getting wet and I figured she could use some fresh air. I started to wheel her toward the door, but she said no, we should go out a different door. The one she wanted had no canopy or overhang. I told her we couldn't go out there because it was raining and she couldn't risk getting her head wet.

No, she insisted, we had to go out that door. When I asked why, she said an airplane was about to crash into the building and we needed to get outside. I wheeled her over to the door where she could look out to see there wasn't anything flying around. That seemed to calm her enough for me to get her back to her room, but she was still anxious about the airplane, so I went to the window to open the blinds and show her there was nothing there. Fortunately, I looked out first, because of course there was an airplane and of course it was flying directly toward the hospital. I closed the blinds and lied to her, reflecting that if the plane did crash into the building, I'd never live it down.

Once we were able to drop her Sinemet to its former level, her hallucinations of disasters and catastrophes disappeared. But our house is still filled with imaginary people and pets, and sometimes she awakens in the morning insisting we get up because it's time to leave the boat or the airplane or whatever craft she imagines we're on.

## Progress and Regress

In 2010, Sandra's stimulator battery expired and she had to have a replacement. Dr. Honey told us she would be getting the new, updated, super-duper, handy-dandy model with its state of the art high-tech controller. (That's not a quote, but the sentiment was there.) The new stimulator was slimmer so it wouldn't be as obtrusive in her chest, and the controller was far more capable than the Stone Age model we'd been using.

However, after the surgery, we learned that the new stimulator wouldn't work with the electrodes in her brain, so it needed an adapter. The combination of adapter and stimulator was thicker than the previous stimulator, so it stuck out from her chest even more than the original had.

But it was the controller—the device that operated the stimulator—that perplexed me. The previous one had been simple. Did we want to adjust the stimulation, either up or down? Just press two buttons: one for each side of the brain. It was so simple that if Sandra wanted an adjustment at night, I could grope for it on my bedside table and work it without even opening my eyes. It was so simple that I was able to make up a one-page instruction sheet for care aides or the staff in a respite home to follow.

Then I met the new controller. And I met the twenty-minute DVD demonstrating its use. And I met the hundred-page manual that came with it. With this new stimulator, I have to press buttons seven times and read a screen. Sometimes it shows a symbol that I guess means something to the designers but is baffling to me. It's probably somewhere in the manual.

When I need to adjust her settings at night, I have to wake up, turn on a light, and read the screen. And preparing instructions for care aides? Describing the income tax code is simpler.

I suppose as technology advances, we have to get even smarter at using it. Like television remotes, things are getting more, not less, complicated, but that's not what we were promised.

I sent the manufacturer a letter thanking them for providing me with an example of poor product usability for my course in quality management. They never wrote back.

# 1 3

# Fighting the Good Fight

Throughout her career, Sandra had always been a fighter. To her, discussions of problems were pointless unless they were aimed at taking action. Early in our marriage, she came home from work at the hospital and said, "I've just been elected shop steward on the ward."

I said, "Who are you and what have you done with my wife?"

Neither of us had ever been union supporters. I'd never belonged to one, and Sandra had joined only because nursing at a public institution in British Columbia required it. But on her ward, things needed shaking up.

One of the nurses was entitled to a benefit on the basis of seniority and, in Sandra's mind, competence, but the head nurse had granted the benefit to a less deserving staff member. Sandra knew why and she was not happy: the nurse who was turned down was a man. Not only that, but he was self-effacing and not inclined to make a fuss. When he told Sandra what had happened, she suggested he talk to the shop steward. According to the collective agreement, he was entitled to the benefit, so the union could intervene on his behalf. But the shop steward was not prepared to help him, probably because she was about to step down and wasn't willing to start another fight.

On the ward, Sandra was vocal about how this man had been deprived of the benefit he had earned. So when the existing shop steward resigned, her colleagues rewarded—or punished—her persistence by electing her. She was the unanimous choice.

Armed with the collective agreement, she told the head nurse either to grant the benefit to the man or prepare for a grievance. The head nurse postured, protested, and then, as if it were her own idea, relented.

Over the next year, Sandra absorbed the collective agreement. She learned that contracts were more effective than indignation in forcing her management to behave. She loved the ability to make sure the contract was honored, and she reveled in being a thorn in this head nurse's side. To be fair, she also spiked complaints from the staff when they demanded benefits the contract didn't cover. Nevertheless, when she stepped down, I suspect the head nurse held a party.

Sandra brought that attitude to her fight against Parkinson's. One incident stands out for me. We had just flown in to Vancouver from a trip outside the country. Sandra hadn't reached the point where she would accept a wheelchair in the airport, but she walked slowly, she needed to rest often, and airports are big.

We reached the escalator down into the customs area. And I groaned. Several jumbo jets had arrived at about the same time, and the hall, half the size of a football field, was almost full with two queues of passengers snaking along between ropes strung from pylons. I suggested to Sandra that I look for a wheelchair, but she said no. When I told her it would probably take half an hour to get through the line, she insisted she could do it. So we joined the queue for Canadian passport holders and began to shuffle along.

After about ten minutes, she was struggling. Each step was an effort for her, and I had to hold on to both her hands to support her. Once again, I suggested a wheelchair; once again she said no—she would finish this. So we continued on. Then I began to hear some comments from a small group a short distance ahead of us. They were tut-tutting about how this poor woman was being made to endure this line and how she should be in a wheelchair. They never spoke to us directly, but their voices became louder and more strident, announcing to all within earshot how much they disapproved of what was happening and, annoying to me, of my role in forcing this unfortunate woman to suffer.

Then a police officer appeared beside us. The group had pointed us out to him. He said he'd get a wheelchair for Sandra. I looked at her, but she shook her head. I told the cop she didn't want one. When he insisted, I told him she saw dealing with this line as a challenge: she was adamant it wouldn't defeat her and she was determined to overcome it. I heard one of the people say oh, just as I barked that her struggle would be a lot easier if some loud-mouthed busybodies would keep their opinions to themselves. The cop looked at us, nodded, and walked off. These people never said another word. I hope the immigration officers gave them a rough time. And if you're tempted to criticize my response on the grounds that these people were just concerned for Sandra's well-being, I disagree. If they had been, they'd have approached me to see if I wanted help or to ask if they could round up a wheelchair for her. Instead, they preferred to advertise to everyone around them how empathetic they were and what good people this made them.

When we got through immigration and into the baggage area, she collapsed into a seat, grinned, and said, "I did it."

"You did. Congratulations. But there wouldn't have been any shame in letting the cop get you a wheelchair."

Her face took on a look I had become accustomed to: she would not tolerate blockheads. She said, "I wasn't going to give those people the satisfaction."

Her words reminded me of my mother, an English war bride who, just after the Second World War, left her home in London to travel to far-off, remote central British Columbia. Before she left, a family acquaintance scoffed that she'd never last; she'd be back in six months. My mother later said those six months were brutal and she often considered giving in and returning to England, but her acquaintance's words always stopped her. She said, "I wasn't going to give her the satisfaction." Here's to strong-willed women.

When I've told Sandra's airport story, some people have commented that her reaction was false pride. They're half right. It was pride, but false is a judgment they're not entitled to make.

Having proven she could conquer airports, Sandra finally relented and began to use a wheelchair when we traveled.

From this incident, I have a request. If you see someone who is struggling, please don't make assumptions. If you are so moved, ask the person if he or she wants (not needs) some help, then respect the answer. I've learned to follow this advice. Sometimes when I offer help, the person accepts with gratitude. Other times he or she says no thanks and sometimes just a blunt no. It's that person's life; I am but an interruption.

# 14

# Are You Senile?

During Sandra's battle with Parkinson's, we became aware of the "Are you senile?" tests that many doctors use. These are questions such as "What is today's date?" or "Do you know where you are?" Apparently it's wrong to answer "Do I look like a calendar?" or "The same place you are." They're trying to assess your mental capability, and the questions they ask sound so reasonable. After all, who doesn't know the date?

Well, how about me? When I worked in an office, the date was at the front of my mind. My day was filled with meetings or deadlines, and my online schedule was prominent on my desktop screen. The date was obvious, and anyone who didn't know it needed help. And of course, the calendar held promise of the important things: weekends and paydays.

Then I began to work at home, focusing on teaching and writing. Except for the days I was supposed to be standing in front of a classroom or meeting a client, the date seemed to lose its importance. Sandra and I still observe the weekends, but I couldn't tell you the date without looking it up.

And there's the problem. The doctors who are asking the question are working to a schedule. They know the date just as much as anyone else in a similar position. When they retire from their practices, they too will find that the date is no longer important, but in the meantime, anyone who doesn't know it is on a downhill slide and will soon be on the floor trying to re-arrange the patterns in the carpet. I've pointed out that the date is only important to those who are working, like they are. They acknowledge what I'm saying, but they still ask the question and they still make notes on the answer.

So my advice is to do what Sandra and I do. Whenever she's going to an appointment, I tell her the date and have her practice so she can answer the question when it comes up.

There are two more tests that some doctors love to administer. One is to spell "world" backward. Memorize "dlrow" so you can ace that test. But don't be too smooth; the doctor will know you practiced.

The other test is to count backward from one hundred by seven—without using a calculator. Subtracting seven from any number where the units digit is less than seven is tricky, but those of us in the know never subtract seven, we subtract ten and add three. Try it. One hundred minus ten is ninety plus three is ninety-three. Once more, ninety-three minus ten is eighty-three plus three is eighty-six. It works. Practice it, but again, give some pretense that you're struggling.

And if you're concerned that all of this is cheating, don't worry. If you can manage these tips, there's nothing wrong with your cognition.

## I Can't Recall the Word

I realized Sandra was starting to have cognitive problems when she couldn't recall common words. At first, I put it down to normal mental glitches or even to aging, when difficulties in finding words often get worse—although I believe this isn't because of some mental decline but because they've got more words stuffed into their brains and it takes longer to look them up. But Sandra was having the problem more and more often, and the words she couldn't remember were becoming simpler. One evening as I was helping her get ready for bed, she asked for "puree." I had no idea what she meant. "You know, puree," she insisted. I said I didn't know. I knew what puree was, but I doubted she wanted creamed broccoli. Then she said, "You know, for the bathroom."

She occasionally took a glass of prune juice for regularity just before bed, so making a wild guess, I said, "Do you mean prune juice?"

"Yes, that's what I said. Puree."

After that, whenever she asked for puree, I would get her some prune juice. Then, sometime later as I was helping her get ready for bed, it was obvious she wanted something, but all she could say was "sheep."

I said, "Sheep? You mean those woolly animals?"

She said, "Yes, sheep."

Now I was flummoxed, and the more confused I became, the more frustrated she was. Then, because she was getting ready for bed, I took a stab and said, "Do you mean prune juice?"

That's what she meant. I can understand "puree." After all, prune juice could be thought of as pureed prunes. But sheep? I still don't understand the connection, and when I asked her about it, she saw how curious it was, but she didn't have an explanation.

Throughout all of this, Sandra's memory has remained acute. She can remember events that happened years ago or hours ago. If I want to recall the name of someone from our past, I'll ask her and she'll usually have the answer. But some aspects of her cognition were declining, as I found out on a day that shook me.

We were in a coffee shop at the mall. This was a routine I insisted on to get her out of the house to some place with bustle and energy. Going out was getting harder because she was often drowsy and minimally responsive, but I felt she needed some stimulation. This day was different. I'd just read an article about something that fascinated me, and I was enthusing about it. Her eyes were alight, she was smiling, and she nodded at the points I made. She was with me. I was delighted. My Sandra was back, and even though I knew it was temporary, it was wonderful.

Then I finished. She smiled and said, "That's really interesting. My husband, Jolyon, would love to hear that."

I didn't know what to say. My only consolation was that she was right.

## Time Can Be Confusing

After that, I began to notice more when her cognition was slipping. I suspect it had been obvious for a long time, but I had been able to avoid acknowledging it. One of her problems was judging time. Vivian was coming to visit us and was due to arrive on Friday. On Tuesday morning, Sandra got up early, and when I asked why, she said her sister was coming and she had to get ready. I said indeed Vivian was coming. Three days from now. She said oh and climbed back into bed. On Wednesday and Thursday, the same thing happened. By Friday, she was ready to greet her sister.

So now, every day when she wakes up, I say, "Today is Tuesday" (assuming, of course, it really is Tuesday). "Nothing's happening, we're not going anywhere, and nobody's coming over." Or I'll say something like, "Today is

Tuesday. You have an appointment, but it's not until the afternoon, so you can rest for now." I've found that reminding her each day settles her down and reduces her anxiety. And mine.

## Visual Perception or Why Am I Reaching for Air?

At some point, I got a sudden lesson on the impairment of visual perception. Normally, our vision tells us where things are and how to interact with them. For example, let's say that you want to pick up a mug of hot coffee. If you're like most of us, you just reach out, pick it up, and raise it to your mouth. While you're doing this, you look at the mug but not at your hand. How does your hand know where to go? Your visual perception has told it. But what happens when that becomes impaired?

One day, Sandra reached for a glass of water, but her hand was wide of the glass. She moved her hand until it touched the glass, then she grasped it and raised it to her mouth. But not exactly. The glass touched her cheek, so she moved it over until it was at her mouth. Then she was able to drink.

When she finished and went to put the glass back down, it caught the edge of a plate, and when she let go, it tipped, spilling water over the table. She could see the plate, but she wasn't able to judge where it was in relation to her hand or the glass she was holding. Other times she goes to put a glass down but misses the table entirely.

Since then, I've learned to watch when she picks something up or puts something down and to make sure she's not going to have problems. At times, I'll even take the glass from her hand and set it down for her.

# 15

# Care Providers and Bureaucrats

Sandra declined to the point where I became aware that either I had to give up work outside the home or I needed help looking after her. For caregivers, particularly men, admitting this can be a problem. We're taught to be self-reliant: that it's a sign of weakness to seek help. But when you need it, not seeking it is less an expression of manliness than a sign of obstinacy. Apparently, I had had it drummed into me neither to seek nor to accept help: to look after myself. Sometimes when Sandra and I were going to a local park for a walk and had to cross the street, a helpful motorist would stop to let us pass. My original reaction was unreasonable anger. Did this idiot think I was helpless, a doddering fool who couldn't even get across the street without his stopping? Caregiving has taught me the value of help and the civility of allowing others to give it. I've since mellowed and I now accept that offer with gratitude, but it was a difficult lesson to accept.

Sometimes, I had to leave our house to teach a course during the day. I'd be back in the evening, but Sandra couldn't cope by herself while I was gone. Then I discovered Burnaby Home Care, who sent over a pleasant woman to assess Sandra. She would become Sandra's case manager and the person I called whenever I needed some coverage during the day. She would arrange for care aides to come in and get Sandra dressed, feed her, and make sure she got her medications. Over the next few years, the case manager changed, but I was always pleased at the responsiveness and concern they all brought to the job.

Then things began to slide. Not in terms of care, but in terms of policy. Before I left for the day, I'd prepare food for Sandra and put it in the fridge, and I'd put out her medications in medicine cups on the dining room table.

Each medicine cup sat on a sheet of paper with a printed description of the medications and the time they were to be given. Then the case manager told me there was a new policy: care aides would only give medications if they were in blister packs. We normally get them in bottles, so this was a problem, but the pharmacy said they'd package up a few days' supply for us. It seemed silly to go to all this work for the couple of days I'd be out of the house, but policy is policy.

Then the policy was "updated," which is bureaucrat-speak for "make it more convenient for us, less for you." Now the care aides couldn't give Sandra her medications regardless of how they were packaged. They could only remind her when it was time to take them. Since she had trouble handling a blister pack, this policy was cruel. Fortunately, this meant that I could now revert to putting the medications in medicine cups.

Then the policy changed again. Now the care aides could no longer even remind Sandra to take her medications. It didn't matter how they were packaged, the care aides would have nothing to do with administering or even discussing them. There was an option: home care would give Sandra her medications if we registered for a special program in which approved care aides would come to the house and give her all her medications, all the time, whether or not I was home. She gets medications six times a day, so this program meant having people at our front door that often. I have no idea what that would cost the health care system, but I knew it would be inconvenient to us. How could we go out for coffee or a walk in the park? Since I'm perfectly capable of giving medications when I'm at home, putting Sandra in this program was ridiculous. Furthermore, it was so complex to set up that it wasn't available on a temporary basis, like the few times we needed it. Now I had a problem: how could I ensure that Sandra got her medications on time when I wasn't there? Fortunately, we had sometimes used a private nursing agency.

The care manager for the agency had assessed Sandra previously and had sometimes provided care aides. I had been impressed with her and her services, so I asked her if her care aides would give medications, even if they were in medicine cups. Yes, she replied. Of course they would: it was their job. What a concept. So now, when I'm away for the day, I bring in care aides from the agency to make sure Sandra gets her medications. It's more expensive than the home care program, but I know she is being cared for.

At the suggestion of Sandra's case manager, who seemed as frustrated by the policy as I was, I wrote a letter of complaint to the health authority. I never heard back. I'm not sure why. Perhaps my reference to "addle-brained pencil pushers" had something to do with it.

## You Can't Use That Name

Sandra's first name is Doris, but she goes by Sandra. She always has. I've found that some services are willing to accommodate her. On their records, she is identified as Sandra, but others, particularly those run by the government, seem to be sticklers. I've often called one of these agencies and asked something about Sandra Hallows, only to be told they don't have any such person in their files. I know they do, and I also know that Hallows is not a name so common that they'd have several.

I've argued that many people use their second names, including a former business partner, a childhood friend, and oh yes, my father. It doesn't seem to matter. Doris is the first name on her health care card: Doris is how they'll refer to her.

I could capitulate and recognize the futility of arguing with bureaucrats, but there's a potentially serious problem. Nobody outside a few rigid agencies has ever called her Doris, so she's not used to that name. If she were in hospital or a clinic and somebody referred to her as Doris, it's possible she wouldn't respond, especially if she were sedated or confused. I can imagine scenarios in which a mix-up over names could endanger her, so it baffles and annoys me when officials, hiding behind the authority they have arrogated, insist on calling her by a name she has never used. So whenever I speak to them and they ask, "Do you mean Doris?" I reply, "No, I mean Sandra. Doris is her first name but she is to be called Sandra."

## The Trials and Rewards of Respite Care

In November 2008, I had an assignment to teach a course in New York. I'd been there several times before, and whenever I went, Vivian would come from Saskatoon to care for Sandra or she would go there. But this was demanding on Vivian, and over time, Sandra was reaching the point where she needed too much help for this to be viable, so Burnaby Home Care arranged for her to go into respite. This is a room in a regular nursing home that people can book for short stays. We were both unsure about how this would work out, but she agreed to try it. When I got back, I asked her if she wanted to get some flowers for the staff. She agreed, and we did.

She wasn't fond of the respite home. She said she would tolerate it, but only just, and after a second stay, she liked it even less. So when I was booked to teach some courses in Manila, her case manager got her a bed in a different home. This place seemed wonderful. It was new. It had flowers and gardens and the foyer of a grand hotel and cheerful staff who boasted of their rehab and exercise programs. This place was clearly better than the previous one, so I was surprised when I picked her up ten days later and asked her if she wanted to get flowers. She glowered at me and snapped, "No. Just get out of here." I later found out that the staff had stuck her in a wheelchair and the ward she was on was locked. She hadn't been allowed out for the entire ten days. No walks in the garden, no rehab, nothing. She never went back.

Her experience there gave her a more favorable attitude toward the original respite home, but when we happened to drive by one day, we saw it had been torn down. I have to say this is a recurring theme in Sandra's history. The Calgary General Hospital, where she trained, no longer exists. The Holy Cross Hospital in Calgary, where she first worked, is no longer a hospital. Riverview Hospital, the B.C. psychiatric hospital where she worked, is closed. Northwestern Hospital in Toronto, where she worked, has been torn down. St. Vincent's Hospital, where she had her medications adjusted, is now a residential care home. I once suggested she should get hospitals to pay her not to work or stay there. The bulldozing of the respite home just continued the pattern.

Then, when I had another trip to New York, her case manager referred her to a care center called Queen's Park Hospital. They had set up a facility dedicated to respite and named it the Respite Hotel. It was new; she was its first guest. When I returned from my trip and picked her up, I hesitated before asking her if she wanted to get flowers for the staff, but she said yes. And chocolates. Since then, she has stayed at the Respite Hotel several times, and I have always been impressed by the care, concern, and professionalism of the staff. Not only that, but when I pick her up, she seems brighter.

# The Day Program

One other service has helped her. I was getting concerned that her world had shrunk down to our house and me. We go out for coffee to a café in a local mall most days. Sometimes I have to push her to go, but it's good for her to get out of the house and be exposed to some action, even if it's the chaos of a mall.

But I wanted outside contact for her where she could interact with others, so her case manager arranged for her to attend an adult day program called Cranberry Cottage. I drop her off at about 10:00 a.m. and pick her up at 3:30. They have lunch, snacks, and activities, she gets to associate with others, and they look after her, including giving her the medications she needs.

When she started going to the program, she resisted. Sometimes when I roused her from her bed, she moaned that she didn't want to go. But each time I picked her up, she was brighter and more alert, so I knew it was benefiting her and I insisted she go. It was also benefiting me. I was able to spend a couple of hours on a nearby par-three golf course, something I'd had to give up when Sandra's disease prevented her from playing.

After a few sessions, I asked her if she'd like to go a second day in the week. Her abrupt no made her position clear, so I didn't broach it again. Then Manjit Deogan, the engaging coordinator, asked if Sandra would like to go on a second day. A vacancy had come up. When I asked Sandra, I got the same curt response. But on the following Saturday, when I woke her for her ten o'clock medications, she asked what time it was. When I told her, she said, "Oh, it's too late."

"Too late for what?" I asked.

"For Cranberry Cottage."

I held my breath. "Do you want to go a second day?"

"Okay."

So I called Manjit and registered her. Now she goes twice a week. I suppose she needed some time to get used to it because she no longer resists going, and whenever I pick her up and ask if she's had a good day, she says she did.

On at least one of her days, I've made a habit of not going home. I wander, shop, sometimes visit colleagues, and usually find an appealing (and sometimes appalling) place for lunch. Then in the afternoon, I'm always glad to see her again.

# 16

# Other Medical Problems

People with Parkinson's, no less than anyone else, can suffer from medical problems other than the disease. For Sandra, one of the annoying outcomes of her diagnosis was that some practitioners blamed Parkinson's for any of her symptoms. One day she said, "Parkinson's is a wonderful disease. Apparently, having it makes it impossible to get anything else."

When she had sore feet, I suggested she see a podiatrist who had seemed to me to be friendly and competent. She said, "He'll just say it's because of my Parkinson's." I assured her he was one of the good guys and would give her a fair examination. Her grimace when she left his office told me otherwise. We were able to find another podiatrist who actually looked at her feet and recommended different shoes.

Of course, Parkinson's doesn't immunize people against other conditions, and for most people, those begin to develop more frequently as they age.

## Osteoporosis

One of Sandra's problems was osteoporosis. Her mother had it badly, and I could see Sandra slowly developing a slouch and a curve in her back. In January 2004, a bone density scan confirmed the condition. She tried the standard treatments such as Fosamax (alendronate), but the side effects of this and similar medications include heartburn and nausea, and she had them both.

Then Dr. Frame referred her to a clinic specializing in, among other things, bone diseases including osteoporosis. To the clinic's doctor, Sandra's reaction to the standard medications was not unusual, and he recommended an alternative: Aclasta, a medication given intravenously and just once a year. Aclasta doesn't build bones, but the doctor expected it would prevent any further deterioration. Visiting the clinic annually also meant that the bone density tests would be given by the same person using the same equipment, reducing variations in the results.

But administering the Aclasta was a problem. Sandra has very fine veins. Many times, I've watched nurses struggle to find one, sometimes needing several attempts by several nurses before they succeed. (By contrast, the technicians at the local medical lab have no problem in hitting a vein on the first try. When I commented on this, the lab tech said she does this dozens of times a day whereas a nurse in a hospital may do it only a few times a week. Practice does make perfect. Or at least better.)

So the staff at the clinic found it hard to hit a vein, and by the time they'd finally succeeded, both they and Sandra were wiped out. So in 2011, her doctor switched her to Prolia, a medication just as effective as Aclasta but given by injection twice a year. Now she could simply go to her family doctor's office, and because the price was spread over two payments, it was easier to bear. And the treatments, either Aclasta or Prolia, worked. Her bone density held steady.

## I Gotta Go – Again

One of the more stressful of Sandra's symptoms was that she had to go to the bathroom at night, sometimes five or six times. We have a bedside commode, but because she couldn't get to it without help, I was also up five or six times a night. On the grounds that this isn't normal, Dr. Frame referred her to the frankly named Bladder Care Centre at the University of B.C. hospital, where in late 2007, we met the Centre's research director, who had the aura of a down-home country doctor with all the time in the world to talk to her patients and maybe even go fishing. At the same time, she was in control of an array of high-tech equipment that measured all aspects of what happens when we go.

That equipment told her Sandra wasn't completely emptying her bladder, which meant not only would she have to go more often, but she was prone to bladder infections. To most people, these are a nuisance, but to

Sandra they can be debilitating. So now when she's feeling out of sorts, we take a urine sample.

Taking a urine sample sounds simple, but I'm convinced that specimen bottles were designed by and for men. They're easy for us to use. For women, not so much, and particularly so for Sandra, who has difficulty telling where her hand actually is. So we were able to sneak off from the Centre with what we call a "hat." It's a plastic container that looks like, well, a hat. It goes under the toilet seat—upside down, of course—and catches the urine, which I can then pour through a handy channel into a specimen bottle. I believe these are intended for single use because I'm sure re-using them doesn't reach hospital standards of sterility. But since I refuse to stand there holding the specimen bottle, Sandra has no alternative.

The clinic's doctor concluded that Sandra probably wouldn't benefit from any of the available treatments, and a new medicine that might have helped hadn't yet been approved by Health Canada.

In the meantime, Sandra had an appointment with Dr. Dian, the geriatrician who had referred her to the St. Vincent's program. He suggested a medication called gabapentin, normally used for epilepsy and pain. Dr. Dian thought it might help her sleep better and, with luck, reduce the frequency with which she had to get up while not inducing night-time accidents.[*] To our gratification, it worked. Under the drug, her frequency dropped to one to three times a night and sometimes not at all. But after a couple of years, night-time accidents started, and I'd noticed that the drug seemed to be making her drowsy. When we stopped it, her nighttime visits to the commode stayed low and have continued to do so. I don't understand why, but I welcome it.

When we discussed Sandra's need to get up so often at night, Dr. Frame suggested she be tested for sleep apnea, a condition in which the sufferer stops breathing at night. He referred Sandra to a clinic at the University of B.C. for an overnight study. This is a gadget-lover's dream. You're covered with stick-on sensors connected to a bank of machines that wouldn't look out of place at a satellite launch. Once you're set up, pasted, and wired, you are told to lie down, relax, and go to sleep. Fat chance. If Sandra had to get up before, this made it even worse. So I slept, or tried to, in an adjacent

---

[*]    A doctor can prescribe a medication for purposes it's not intended for if he or she believes it will help. This is called an "off-label" prescription and it's perfectly legal. However, the manufacturer of the medication can't claim that it's effective for this other purpose.

room, and whenever she had to get up, I'd help her while the nurse would disconnect all of the leads from the bank of machines and, when she was finished, hook them back up.

I'm still tired.

The tests showed she had mild sleep apnea but not enough to worry about. The doctor suggested she elevate her head at night, so we bought a foam rubber wedge that went under the pillow. I got one as well because I'd been having problems with acid reflux, and elevating the head is supposed to help. It worked for me and I suspect it helped Sandra, except that, annoyingly, I now tend to slide down in the bed until my feet are sticking out the end. That wakes me up even more than Sandra's nocturnal needs.

## Peripheral Vision

I was getting concerned about Sandra's vision. At times, she couldn't see things that were clearly in front of her. Her eye tests all came back normal. She had always worn glasses and her prescription got a little stronger, but that's common with aging. Yet there were times when I doubted her test results.

So Dr. Frame referred her to a neuro-ophthalmologist. I'd always been impressed by the array of machines that ophthalmologists use, but this office was unlike any I'd ever seen: a baffling combination of high-tech equipment alongside stuffed toys and rubber ducks. Some of her tests were familiar—reading letters projected onto a wall—while others were unusual. One involved looking into a large circular bowl as a light popped up randomly around it. The results were not encouraging: Sandra had lost most of her peripheral vision. She could see things in front of her, but those to the side had become invisible.

The ophthalmologist consulted with Dr. Honey, speculating that the placement of the DBS electrodes was interfering with the visual pathways, but a scan of Sandra's brain indicated otherwise. The good news was that the condition didn't appear to be getting worse.

So now, I make sure everything she needs is directly in front of her.

# 17

# Once More at the University

In 2011, I was getting concerned about the amount of sleep Sandra needed. She'd go to bed before 10:00 p.m. and wouldn't get up until noon or later. Her family doctor suggested she consult the Pacific Parkinson's Research Centre at the University of B.C. This was the successor of the Movement Disorders Centre we had rejected years earlier, but on the grounds that people, and sometimes institutions, change, we decided to give it another try. The staff were thorough; several specialists examined Sandra over about three hours before she was finally seen by one of the Centre's neurologists. At the time, she was taking Sinemet and pramipexole. The doctor spent about five minutes with us before she suggested phasing out the pramipexole. Then she said, "I'll see you in eight months."

Eight months? Stop taking a potent medication without some sort of monitoring? We were not impressed. Nevertheless, Sandra began reducing her pramipexole dosage. It made no difference to her sleep habits.

Eight months later, we returned to the UBC Centre. Once again, Sandra spent three hours being tested, probed, and analyzed, and once again, she had no more than a few minutes with the neurologist, who this time suggested she drink caffeinated coffee to help her stay awake. Not only had we already tried this, but the advice didn't seem to warrant all of the testing they were doing. I began to wonder why these people got the big bucks. Driving home after we left the clinic, I could see that Sandra was exhausted, but worse, disheartened. These tests made it obvious to her how much she had declined and how little she could do for herself. For example, one of the examiners asked her to draw a shape that looked like a house. Sandra's efforts bore no resemblance to the original. Of course, she could see what she drew, and the results dismayed her. If all of this had helped, we might have tolerated it, but the value of her visits to the Centre was close to zero.

Nine months later, I got a call from the Centre reminding us of an appointment the following day. I hadn't known we had an appointment and we couldn't make it. When I asked the receptionist to re-book it, she did—fourteen months into the future. They made no attempt to accommodate their slipup in failing to let me know of the appointment, but I figured when you're only concerned with collecting data, time probably doesn't matter as much.

Then things changed. Remarkably so.

Sandra and I had dismissed the Centre as having any value for her. We decided to skip the next appointment, but we left it open just in case we changed our minds. And it was fortunate we did.

From my Parkinson's caregivers support group, I heard of a doctor at UBC whom several people raved about but who was hard to get in to see. So when the appointment at the UBC Centre came up, we decided to go for no other reason than to ask for a referral.

We were expecting a repeat of the previous two visits, but to our surprise, that didn't happen. The Centre had moved into a new building. Whether this lifted the spirits of the people there I'm not sure, but the attitude was completely different. Instead of the intimidating round of tests we'd expected, we sat down with a neurological fellow who strolled with us through a questionnaire. There was no rush; we could take our time. Then we saw one of the Centre's neurologists, who consulted with us for almost twenty minutes. She noted Sandra's symptoms and prepared a plan to deal with them. She added a new medication and reduced the frequency of another. She recommended therapies for other problems. She also agreed to provide the referral we'd asked for. When Sandra and I left, we looked at one another and wondered what had just happened.

The referral was to Andrew Howard, a neuropsychiatrist. Neuropsychiatry is a medical specialty combining neurology and psychiatry. Dr. Howard booked three hour-long sessions, his examinations impressing both of us. Then he said he wanted to try some different medications, but only one at a time. We have since seen him several times. As a result, Sandra now takes three other medications, all of which have improved her function. The first time we saw him, he said he wished he'd seen her sooner in the course of her disease. I did too.

He also brings out the best in her. During one examination, she was having a bad day. She was unresponsive and unable to answer the simplest of questions. When he asked her to repeat 2-1-8, she could do so, but she couldn't say the numbers backward. He finished his examination, leaned toward her, held her hands, looked into her eyes, and said, "How are your spirits?" Without any change in her demeanor, she said, "They're still in the bottle."

He gaped at her and said, "They're still in the bottle?" Then he looked at me and my stunned expression, and all three of us began laughing. When we left with a new prescription, he said any improvement would be small, perhaps five percent. I said twenty medications at five percent each and we're there!

# 18

# The Wilfrid Laurier Program

In 2010, I learned of a Parkinson's exercise rehabilitation program at Wilfrid Laurier University in Waterloo, Ontario. The results sounded impressive, and because it was experimental, it was free. But it ran for three months.*

Waterloo is about four thousand kilometers (twenty-five hundred miles for the non-metric) from Burnaby, so this would be a major commitment. We decided to go for it. In early September 2010, we packed our car and drove east.

The program was run by Wilfrid Laurier University's Sun Life Movement Disorders Research & Rehabilitation Centre, a mouthful they condensed down to "MDRC." The Centre's director, Quincy Almeida, isn't a medical doctor; his specialty is kinesiology: the science of human movement. He and his Centre focus on research into Parkinson's. While the descriptions of the program were enough to get us to commit to the trip, encountering it in person was even more impressive.

The program was unusual in two respects. First, all participants were paired with kinesiology students who remained with them for the entire program. So Sandra's volunteer, Rebecca, a cheerful and enthusiastic Laurier student, got to know her and how she moved and was able to help her far more than someone who only saw her once or twice.

Second, the program covered the gamut of therapies for the disease, including exaggerated walking, chair exercises, and voice exercises. I wanted to watch, but since the program was experimental, the work they did was proprietary. Once the participants were inside, they closed the

---

* Laurier. Contact information is available on their website.

door. I understood their concern: there was nothing to prevent me from documenting the exercises and selling them as my own. Furthermore, they couldn't know if I was the type of person who had a lawyer on speed dial who would be my first call if Sandra fell and broke something while I was leading her in one of their exercises. So once I dropped Sandra off, I headed to a nearby coffee shop.

The program was one hour, three times a week for three months. We found a furnished apartment and became residents of Southern Ontario, which enabled us to reconnect with some great friends as well as take in some of the sights.

When the program ended in mid-December, we re-packed the car and headed west. Our trip to Waterloo had been gentle: we took ten days. This time, we just wanted to get home as fast as possible, so we took the route through the U.S., driving across Michigan, northern Indiana, Illinois, Iowa, Nebraska, Wyoming, Utah, Idaho, Oregon, and Washington, back to B.C. We left Waterloo on a Friday afternoon and pulled into our home the following Tuesday just before midnight. This wasn't the shortest route, but it was more southerly and, according to the weather reports that I monitored up to the last minute, warmer. We did hit the corner of a blizzard near Des Moines, but had we taken the more northerly route, we'd have hit the main storm: one that made the evening news in two countries. I suspect we'd still be in a ditch somewhere in Minnesota. My foresight also paid off: before we left Burnaby, I had installed snow tires on the car, knowing it would be winter when we returned. Since that was in September, the garage in Vancouver thought I was mad.

And did all of this work for Sandra?

Yes, it did. Her UPDRS score was taken before and after the program, and at the end, she had dropped fourteen points. Remember, lower is better. The average difference in UPDRS scores between a person's "on" and "off" states is seven to eight points,* so fourteen was the equivalent of reversing several years of decline.

There was one other change for which I am thankful. Before she took the program, she couldn't get onto a down escalator. Up was okay, but not down. If we had to go down, we had to search for an elevator or struggle down a staircase. Then, during the program, we were in a mall, and without thinking she got on one. To this day, she is still able to ride it. Sometimes

---

*    Bordelon.

getting on is a struggle, but she can do it. The first time she stepped onto the escalator, I said, "You're an old pro."

She scowled and said, "I'm not old."

She didn't seem any happier when I said, "Young amateur?"

# 19

# Independence and Its Decline

## The End of Driving

Sandra always valued her independence and our travels, but her Parkinson's brought those to a close. Toward the end of 2004, she went in to renew her driver's license. The clerk, noticing that she was having problems, ordered a driver's test. By this time, Sandra's ability to respond to the world around her was diminishing and her judgment was declining. She failed the test. I took her out for lessons and found out why the experts recommend having a professional teach driving. All I can say is that's not a job I'd be good at. So, to give her the best chance, she took lessons from a driving school.

She failed her second test, so in January 2005, the Motor Vehicle Branch pulled her license. I found her sitting in a chair in tears, the letter in her lap. It was the only time I ever saw her cry because of the disease. And it was one of the few times I felt like a cad, because even as I held her and joined in her condemnation of petty bureaucrats, I knew they had made the right decision.

## The End of Traveling

We were able to make the trip to Waterloo in part because Sandra had always loved to travel. Even after she became more disabled, she would sometimes accompany me on a business trip. She came to New York City with me a couple of times, and in the late summer, we often went to Marlborough, Massachusetts, for the annual convention of the National Guild of Hypnotists. On our last such trip, we drove from New York through Connecticut and Rhode Island to Massachusetts with a side trip up Cape Cod.

Whenever we left Canada, we'd arrange for travel medical insurance. The first time I bought insurance after Sandra was diagnosed, I braced myself for sticker shock: this would be expensive. To my astonishment, the cost for me was higher than for her. My only chronic medical condition is high blood pressure, which I've controlled for years with pills. But that was enough to bump me into a higher category. Parkinson's wasn't even on the endless list of ailments the insurance company asked about. (I recommend reading such a list. No matter how sick you are, identifying the conditions you don't have can be a tonic.)

Her longest trip was to Manila. After I finished my assignment, we went for a week to the Filipino resort of Boracay, where we lounged on a vast sand beach and alternated between Filipino beer and mango shakes. In a café in Manila, we heard the unmistakable voice of Bing Crosby singing "I'm Dreaming of a White Christmas." It was September and thirty degrees Celsius—over eighty degrees Fahrenheit—so it seemed to be out of place. When I mentioned this to my client, he said Filipinos celebrate Christmas during the "ber" months. When I looked at him quizzically, he said, "September, October, November, and December." I replied that in Canada, the ber months were December to February. When he looked at me quizzically, I shivered and said, "brr."

But her traveling days were coming to an end. I realized this in a big way in the summer of 2011. Sandra had received a note from her longtime friend Della Bascom, one of her classmates in the nursing program and her maid of honor. They had kept in touch over the years, so when the psychiatric hospital in Ponoka was celebrating its hundredth anniversary, Sandra said she wanted to go. We decided to make a vacation of it, so in mid-July we drove across southern B.C. and Alberta, spending a night at a hot springs and stopping at the delightfully named Head-Smashed-In Buffalo Jump and the Royal Tyrell Museum, with its astonishing collection of dinosaurs and other extinct creatures. We continued on to Saskatoon, where we spent some time with Vivian and visited friends and family, then headed to Ponoka for the party. We spent three days there, mostly visiting classmates whom Sandra hadn't seen since 1967. When the party ended, we left to return to B.C.

I'd noticed that all of this travel was taking its toll on her. She was getting less and less responsive and spent most of the time nodding off even as she was visiting her former classmates. On our way home, we'd planned to swing by Penticton to visit Nick and Bev, and the first night heading back, we arrived at the town of Golden.

I pulled into a motel, but the only vacancy was on an upper floor and they didn't have an elevator. When I returned to the car, Sandra's door was open and she was sitting on the seat with her feet on the ground. I said, "Might as well get back in the car. They don't have a vacancy."

She protested that of course they did and we were staying here tonight. I said we couldn't, but there were lots of motels in town and we'd find another one. By now, she was in tears, struggling to stand up and getting more and more distressed. She said, "We'll talk to the manager. He'll get us a room."

She refused to get back in the car, so I got in the driver's side, expecting that once I was ready to drive away she'd relent. She didn't. She was crying and agitated, insisting that we stay in that motel. So I went around to her door, forced her legs back into the car while she struggled, then closed and locked the door and got into my side. She was upset, crying, and trying to open her door, but the minute I started to pull away, she settled down. I don't know what she had seen that set her off, but once we pulled out of the parking lot, she was fine.

I found another motel, registered, and was walking back to the car when a woman's voice boomed out from the sky, "Step away from the car."

I looked back toward the motel office but couldn't see anything, and I wasn't even sure that the order was meant for me. But when I moved forward, the voice again commanded, "Step away from the car."

Then I saw a police cruiser, lights flashing, parked a short distance behind me.

Now I admit to being an aggressive driver. It's one of my responsibilities. People who take defensive driving courses need offensive drivers on whom to practice their skills. That's my role. So I wondered what inattentive infraction could have caused this kerfuffle.

Then a second cruiser pulled up, lights on, and two police officers got out and walked up to me. The woman who had ordered me away from the car said, "We have a report of physical abuse."

Someone had seen me forcing Sandra into the car and had called the cops.

I explained to her what had happened just as a third cruiser pulled up. Then she said, "Stay here," and went over to my car, opened Sandra's door, and started talking to her.

When a fourth cruiser pulled up, I said to the officer standing beside me, "Isn't this a little overkill?" He was pleasant, friendly, and armed. He said, "We respond in force to this kind of complaint." He wasn't kidding. I was waiting for the SWAT team and the helicopters.

The police officer talked to Sandra for about ten minutes, then came back and said, "I'm satisfied with the explanation. We won't be laying any charges." She smiled and said something about how they're taught to treat older people as they'd like their grandparents to be treated. Then she got back in her car and the cruisers pulled out.

I expected the motel owner to come out screaming that he didn't want our type staying at his place, but when nobody appeared, I got back in the car, drove to our room, settled Sandra in bed, and headed for the motel's hot tub for the soak I figured I'd earned.

Then it began to sink in. They weren't going to lay charges. Charges! I was one cop's judgment away from a criminal record, from a restraining order, from being barred from seeing my wife without supervision. I started to shake. I was able to calm myself long enough to call Nick, tell him what had happened, and let him know we were heading home the next day and wouldn't be visiting. When I hung up, my brother's shock and support still roiling in my head, I had to fight not to break down.

The next day, we drove straight back to Burnaby. My despair and frustration had turned to anger, to rage. I was furious at the feebleminded, pinheaded, half-witted moron who had called the cops, who had dared to accuse me of abuse. I understood at a gut level why the police keep such complaints confidential because I itched to get my hands around the neck of whoever had done this. How could this be? Reporting me! I'd made it my life to care for Sandra. How dare anyone say I'd abused her?

And yet . . .

Abuse happens. Too often, the news media report on children or the elderly who have been starved, beaten, and sometimes murdered by those who are supposed to be looking after them. And someone else usually knew of the abuse and did nothing about it.

So here is my request. If you see something that looks like abuse, report it. The police will keep your name confidential and you won't be required to testify in any trial. So report it. And if the person you report turns out to be me, I will be outraged.

Report it anyway.

Sandra had just two more trips. The following summer, Vivian had a milestone birthday and her sons held a surprise party for her, so we flew to Saskatoon for the event. And later we drove to Penticton to visit Nick and Bev. On both trips, I could see her fading after just two or three days. She was less responsive, and at the same time she was becoming more anxious. So we no longer travel. That phase of our lives has ended.

# 20

# There Is a Future

Today as I write this, it's late 2015. Christmas decorations adorn the stores and the days are getting shorter. I have accepted my role as caregiver and what it means. I do all the shopping, the cooking, and the dishes. I do the laundry and the ironing, the vacuuming and the sweeping. I'd make someone a great wife.

I also look after Sandra, which means she's fed and has clean clothes—including her bra, which I have now mastered—she's safe, and she has her medications. I noticed she sometimes put her shoes on the wrong feet. When I pointed this out, she laughed and made some comment. She liked it when I said, "Hey, turkey, now you put your socks on the wrong feet."

But just as much as I look after her physical security, I have become protective of her mental well-being. The years haven't been kind to Sandra. Her osteoporosis has stooped her back, and her Parkinson's has given her a shuffling walk and a flat facial expression; she looks older than she is. Sometimes strangers have referred to her as my mother. If Sandra isn't with me, I'm polite when I correct them, but if she is, I am blunt and unkind. I know they didn't mean to offend her, but they did and I don't forgive them for it. She can't defend herself. I can.

I've also learned that the world is full of good, kind people. People who hold the door open for us—even when it's automatic. People who offer her a seat—even when there are some available. And one woman whose act of kindness still chokes me up.

Christmas was approaching and Sandra and I were at our favorite coffee shop. It's in the mall, with chairs and tables outside the store where we can relax and enjoy the bustle. A young woman, pushing a baby in a stroller, came up to us and handed me two red carnations wrapped in clear plastic and tied with a ribbon. At first, I thought she was selling them or collecting money for some Christmas charity, but she said she'd seen us around and wanted to give us the flowers. I thanked her, we exchanged Christmas greetings, and she walked away. I never found out who she was, but I read the handwritten card she had taped to the plastic: "You are the true love. I see the true love."

Those carnations have died, but we always replace them with fresh ones, and the note will always be with us.

Like all of us, Sandra has good days and not-so-good days. Unlike most of us, the difference between them is stark.

On her good days, she talks, she laughs, she jokes, and she is engaged. On the others, she is almost like an automaton. She has difficulty even opening her eyes, she is hard to maneuver, and she spends most of her time in bed. On good days, she takes her medications without question or difficulty. On her poor days, I have to insist, sometimes force, her to take them.

And it's not even correct to talk about good or poor days, because she can change radically from one hour to the next. Before she was confined to a wheelchair, whenever we went out I had a test to determine how she was going to be. Our house has seven steps from the front door. On some days, she walked down them almost normally, alternating steps. On other days, she clung to the rail and struggled down, one stair at a time, each step an effort, sometimes putting a foot in a place where there was nowhere for the other foot to go.

When I seat her in the car, I hand her the seatbelt. On some days, when I get in she's already buckled up. Other times, she's dropped the seatbelt and I have to find it and manipulate it in place.

I don't know what the future will hold. Even if there is a medical breakthrough, she will still need full care. And if there isn't, she, or I, will reach the stage where I can no longer care for her, and she, or both of us, will need to move into a care home. In the meantime, we live day by day, because there are no other options.

Her good times are welcome and her not-so-good times are a chore. But at night, when I get into bed, sometimes my movements trigger the night light and I lie there watching her sleeping. And sometimes I see the face of a young woman laughing beside a campfire, and the song "Some Enchanted Evening" plays in my head.

# Part III

# Caregiving

# 21

# The Three Dimensions of Caregiving

If you are your loved one's caregiver, this means that as she declines you are responsible to look after her and to make sure she eats, wears clean clothes, takes her medications, bathes, has some form of entertainment, and is safe.

This takes twenty-four hours a day, seven days a week, relieved only by the occasional stay in respite or the attention of care aides. It can break anyone and therefore demands that you take some time to look after yourself. After all, in an airliner, when the oxygen masks drop, you're supposed to put yours on first.

There is an anecdote, exploited by motivational speakers, called the "boiling frog." According to the story, if you put a frog in boiling water, it will jump out, but if you put it in cool or tepid water and gradually heat it, the frog will remain in place until it's cooked. Biologists have debunked this—apparently frogs are smarter than motivational speakers—but the story has become a metaphor for how people slide into behaviors over time that they wouldn't take on all at once. And that describes the progress of caregiving.

With Parkinson's, the changes in your loved one will, in most cases, be gradual, as will the demands on your time and effort. At first, you may simply have to help her get up from a chair. When you go for a walk, holding her hand becomes less a gesture of affection and more a means of support. But over time, you will notice that you have become responsible for helping her with all of the activities of her life. And the changes will have crept up on you in increments, giving you the chance to get accustomed to each one before the next one comes along.

Few of us know how to be caregivers, and aside from training programs for professionals, there are no courses in it. When I reviewed the literature for this book, I was struck by the lack of information for or by caregivers; most of what I found was aimed at patients. Even the websites I found dealt almost exclusively with the emotional side: the anger, grief, despair, and frustration. This was not enough. I agree these are important. But for me, one of the biggest sources of frustration is having to face a problem and not knowing how to deal with it. I wanted something else. I wanted to know how.

So everything I have learned has been from experience, and as writer Steven Wright said, "Experience is something you don't get until just after you need it." My journey would have been easier with some kind of road-map. I hope what I've learned helps you.

I need to make three points. First, while I am the caregiver for my wife, Sandra, not all caregivers look after their spouses. Some care for elderly or infirm parents, some for disabled adult children, and a few for friends or more distant relatives. Much of what I'm saying assumes your loved one is your spouse. If that's not the case, please modify the advice to your personal situation.

Second, a note about the terminology I'll be using. Parkinson's affects both men and women, but "him or her" or "he or she" gets tiresome, and as a writer, I have too much respect for the language to violate its grammar with "they." So in this section, I'll be referring to your loved one as "she." For me, that's true, and as the one who wrote this, I get to choose.

Third, Sandra has Parkinson's, but many caregivers deal with loved ones who have other conditions. If that's true for you, I hope this information helps. Much of caregiving is specific to the disease: medical interventions vary as do symptoms. But much of it is in common. Giving a sponge bath doesn't depend upon the condition. Neither does feeding or hygiene. While I can't comment on the care that depends on the condition, I hope I can help you with its other aspects.

# The Three Dimensions of Caregiving

Caregiving is a mix of physical activities such as giving medications to your loved one or feeding her; installing structural features such as grab bars in the shower or a medical alert system; and dealing with the emotional turmoil that caregiving brings. In the following chapters, I deal with each of these dimensions: physical, structural, and emotional.

Now, I'm sure that some of the pickier readers will say of some activity, "That's not physical, that's structural," or "That activity is both physical and emotional." Disagreement is a risk whenever we try to put anything into categories.* But it doesn't matter where an activity goes, so if it satisfies you to shuffle them around, be my guest. Just don't lose any of them.

# A Word about Professions

You are about to enter a world teeming with people who bring various skills to the care of patients: doctors, of course, but also different types of therapists, nurses, care aides, and others. Let me introduce you to the menagerie of specialists, what each one does, and what you can expect from them.

In the following list, I have included some specialties that overlap or may be confusing. I have not included practitioners of alternative medicine.

- Neurologists are medical doctors who specialize in conditions of the central nervous system, including the brain. Many neurologists don't focus on Parkinson's (although most of them have had to deal with it). Their primary interest may be disorders resulting from brain tumors or head injuries.

- Movement disorder specialists are neurologists who deal with diseases such as Parkinson's that impair movement.

- Physiatrists (note: not psychiatrists) are medical doctors who deal with disorders of the musculoskeletal system, in particular the management of pain.

- Geriatricians *vs.* gerontologists. Geriatricians are medical doctors who specialize in diseases of the elderly. Gerontologists are non-medical specialists who study aspects of aging.

---

\* For example, astronomers quarreled for years over whether Pluto should be categorized as a planet. Pluto lost.

- Psychiatrists *vs.* neuropsychiatrists *vs.* psychologists. Psychiatrists are medical doctors who specialize in disorders of the mind such as dementia or psychoses. Neuropsychiatrists are medical doctors who combine neurology and psychiatry. Psychologists are non-medical professionals who study, among other things, the mind and behavior.

- Physiotherapists *vs.* occupational therapists. There is some overlap here, but broadly, a physiotherapist treats conditions such as injuries or physical disabilities, while an occupational therapist reviews and makes recommendations on the patient's environment, including devices to assist in what they call the "activities of daily living" or ADL.

- Nurses—registered, licensed, practical, and practitioners. The differences between the levels of nursing are those of education and the services the nurse is qualified to provide. Registered nurses (RNs) have the highest level of training and the most responsibilities. In some jurisdictions, nurse practitioners are RNs who have taken advanced courses and are authorized to provide some functions usually restricted to doctors, particularly in remote or small communities. Licensed and practical nurses (LPNs or RPNs) have fewer responsibilities and usually work under more senior nurses.

- Care aides are professionals who provide hands-on care, either in an institution or as part of home services.

# 22

# The Physical Dimension

## The Basics

The physical side of caregiving deals with keeping your loved one safe and clean. It includes preparing meals and feeding her, dressing her, tending to her personal hygiene, and giving her medications. These are the same activities that care aides carry out, but there's one important difference between what they do and what you do.

Care aides usually see their patients as a series of snapshots in time. They're trained to evaluate and respond to the level of care the patients need at that moment. You see your loved one continually when her abilities to look after herself vary from day to day and even from hour to hour. Today, she can cut up her food and feed herself. A few months later, you'll have to do the cutting some of the time, but she can still get the food onto a spoon or fork and move it to her mouth. And several months after that, you'll have to start feeding her too.

And all of this doesn't happen at once. Just like anyone else, your loved one will have good days and bad days, so if you have to cut up her food today, that doesn't mean you'll have to do it again tomorrow.

So giving care means being sensitive to your loved one's needs now.

### Learning from Care Aides

Care aides are trained to provide the basics; it's their job. So you can learn from them. For example, how do they dress a patient and can you pick up any tips? I had been having trouble getting Sandra to put her arm through the sleeve of a blouse or sweatshirt. She would tense her arm and I couldn't get her hand into the armhole. So it was a revelation to me when I watched a care aide dress her. The aide slid her hand down the sleeve from the end, grasped Sandra's hand to extend her arm, and slid the sleeve down. Easy.

So when you have care aides come in, spend some time observing them. Ask questions. After all, they've been to care aide school. You (probably) haven't.

### Offering Help

When you see someone struggle, particularly your loved one, your first inclination is to help. That's not the best strategy because as Sandra once said of a particular care aide, "She hovers." Now, this may seem to contradict what I said earlier about learning from care aides, but remember that, unless you have hired them to come in on a regular basis, they see your loved one briefly and occasionally, then they go home. You're better at assessing what your loved one needs or wants now as opposed to yesterday or a few hours ago.

So this is the approach we worked out: I won't help Sandra unless she asks for it or I can see she's in difficulty. At times, I may ask her if she'd like my help, and I always respect her answer. When I've substituted my judgment for hers and jumped in to help her, she pushed me away. If I complain, "I'm just trying to help," she ignores me. She wants to do it herself and my job is to let her while making sure she doesn't hurt herself.

### Seeing Doctors and Hospitals

One thing I insist on, and Sandra has never questioned, is that I sit in on all of her doctors' appointments. She has never objected, but if she had, I would have seen them separately. I need to know what treatments they prescribe or services they recommend so that I can follow up. I also need to know what Sandra has told them because she sometimes understates her symptoms and overstates her degree of independence. She might not like it, but her doctors need to know the full extent of her condition.

Sandra is prone to falling, and sometimes we've determined that she needs to go to the hospital (although not always: see below under "Falls"). If the emergency room doctor reports that there are no broken bones, I always ask him or her to take a second look. After one fall, she was in a lot of pain. The doctor studied her X-ray and told her she had a soft tissue injury; there were no broken bones. But the pain persisted, so a couple of days later, her family doctor sent her to a radiology clinic for another X-ray. The result: seven fractured ribs. I understand it can be hard to spot a broken rib, perhaps even two. But seven? From that point on, whenever we go to the emergency room, I always insist that the doctor take a second look at the test results. This strategy paid off when Sandra broke her acetabulum. The doctor first reported that nothing was broken. After I insisted he double-check, he came back and said, "It's a good thing I decided to have a second look . . ."

# Taking Care of Your Loved One

### *Personal Hygiene*

Unpleasant though it may be, your loved one's capabilities will decline to the point where she needs help with personal hygiene. This includes not only such activities as brushing her teeth or washing her hands and face, but cleaning after bowel movements.

Get some disposable gloves (non-latex if you or your loved one is allergic to it) and some wet wipes. You'll need them.

Problems can arise when you're not at home. I keep a small pack in our car with latex gloves, wet wipes in individual sachets, a packet of facial tissues, a garbage bag, and a fresh set of panties and slacks. If she has an emergency, I can get her into a handicapped restroom and tend to her, with the soiled clothes going into the garbage bag for laundering.

### *Toilet*

The toilet in our bathroom is awkward to get into. I can maneuver Sandra into it, but care aides had problems, so we came up with this solution.

I installed a small grab bar vertically on the bathroom wall so the bottom of the bar is about three-and-a-half feet from the floor. Now the care aides wheel her into the bathroom and swing the wheelchair so it faces the wall. They help her grip the grab bar and stand up, then they remove the chair, lower her pants, place a commode behind her, and help her sit down on it.

When she's finished, they reverse the procedure. She stands up, then they remove the commode, clean and dress her, and help her back into the wheelchair.

### *Bathing*

This is how I give Sandra a shower. First, I turn on the water so it's hot; I don't want to have frigid water in the tub when she's in it. Then I turn off the water and walk her to the side of the tub. She steps into the tub while holding onto a grab bar. Once there, I maneuver her onto the shower seat.

Once she's seated, I turn on the water to what I think is the right temperature and volume and let her test it. Then I use a hand-held shower head to spray the water over her to wet her down thoroughly, including her hair. Next, I turn off the shower so the water is running through the spout instead of the shower head. I don't want to turn the water off because it would be tricky to get it back to the right temperature. Throughout this procedure, I direct the water through the shower only when I'm rinsing her off. Otherwise, it goes through the spout.

Now I soap and wash her hair, then rinse off the soap. I may repeat this, and when I'm done, I massage conditioner into her hair.

For the next step, I soap a shower pouf and soap her down from her feet to her face. Then I rinse her off, including the conditioner.

Next, I have her stand facing the wall and gripping the grab bar, where I soap her lower back, buttocks, groin, and thighs. Then I rinse off the soap and turn off the water.

While she's still standing, I dry her back, buttocks, and groin, then drape the towel over the shower chair and help her sit down. I finish drying her with another towel, which I then lay on the floor. I help her out of the tub and walk her into the bedroom where I dress her. She walks across the towel so her feet won't slip on the damp floor.

Once she's dressed, I dry her hair with a hair dryer and pretend I'm a hair stylist to get her hair into a semblance of order.

Finally, I rinse off the pouf, clean the tub, and dry the floor with an older towel.

### Giving a Sponge Bath

There may be times when your loved one cannot take a shower or bath. So how do you keep her clean? Give her a sponge bath. Here's how I do it when Sandra can't shower.

I get a basin of hot, mildly soapy water, a face cloth, a towel, and two bath towels. I get her out of the bed and have her stand up or sit on a commode. (If your loved one can't get out of bed, then roll her onto the opposite side.) Then I lay the two bath towels on the bed so they cover one side of it completely from the pillow to the foot. Finally, I get her to lie down on her back on the towels. They protect the sheet from getting wet.

I wet the face cloth and let her wash her face. When she's finished, I give her the towel to dry herself. Of course, I could do this step for her, but I want her to feel she's participating instead of being helpless. And sometimes she asks me to wash her face for her.

Then I wash and dry portions of her body, one at a time, soaking the face cloth after each part. In our bed, she lies on the right-hand side so when I'm washing her, I'm standing on her right. If your bed is the opposite, you can reverse the sides in these instructions, although it doesn't matter.

These are the areas of her body and the sequence in which I wash them.

1. Her right arm, shoulder, and neck, paying particular attention to the armpit and hand.

2. Her left arm, shoulder, and neck, again paying particular attention to the armpit and hand.

3. Her upper chest and both sides, down to her lower abdomen.

4. Her right leg, paying attention to her feet.

5. Her left leg, again paying attention to her feet.

6. Her lower abdomen and groin.

7. Then I roll her onto her left side, facing away from me, and I wash the right side of her back and her right hip and buttock.

8. Next I roll her onto her right side facing me, and I wash the left side of her back and her left hip and buttock.

9. Finally I wash between her buttocks.

10. When I'm finished and while she's still lying on her right side, I roll the towels up and push them under her. Then I roll her back onto her left side and pull the towels out.

11. Finally, I cover her up, let her rest, and clean up the towels, the face cloth, and the basin.

For each of these areas, I wash and dry them thoroughly.

I know that I'll get some reaction from care aides about washing her groin before I do her back. I do it this way because once I've washed her back, I remove the towels; if I washed her anymore, I would risk getting the bed sheet wet.

I also suspect that I'll get some criticism for washing her with soapy water and not rinsing her off before I dry her. But the water is mildly soapy and there's no soap lather on her. Drying her thoroughly will remove any soap residue.

## Dressing

Dressing Sandra was getting to be more and more difficult as her disease progressed. I needed two hands to hold her up and two more to pull up her pants. Since I'm not so endowed, it was a struggle. This is how I do it now.

I move her to the end of the bed and sit her down. It would be easier if she could sit on the side of the bed, but in our bedroom, there's not enough room. I put on her bra and top. Then I put on her panties and pants, pulling them up above her knees. Next, I put on her socks and shoes. With my right hand, I grasp her under her knees and lift her. With my left hand, I maneuver her pants into place. It's still difficult, but it gets the job done.

I also had a problem putting on her slacks because sometimes, particularly if she was restless, I'd end up with her legs in the wrong pant legs, or worse, both legs in one pant leg. So now when I dress her, I hold onto her right pant leg, maneuver her left leg into the other one, then finish up with her right leg. No more problems.

## Eating

Tremors make eating difficult because the food doesn't stay on the utensil. One solution is the children's ditty:

> I eat my peas with honey.
> I've done it all my life.
> It makes the peas taste funny,
> But it keeps them on the knife.

More conventionally, there are utensils adapted to help people with disabilities. Most of them weren't useful for Sandra but that doesn't mean they won't help you. And new products are always being developed. Give them a try.

We found that Sandra could eat soup served in a mug instead of a bowl; she can drink it like a cup of coffee. If it's thin like broth, she can use a straw. Get the kind that bends. If it's a soup with chunky vegetables, I put only the broth in the cup. The vegetables go into a separate bowl so that she can eat them with a fork.

We found a useful device called a "food bumper": a plastic rim that clips to a dinner plate creating a lip that the person can use to push food onto a fork or spoon. It's available from most medical supply stores.

Before her DBS surgery, when tremors made drinking difficult, we used a sealed cup—the kind most coffee stores offer—with a straw. Spilling from that takes talent and resolve.

Sandwiches can be a problem if the contents slide out. The sandwiches I make for Sandra have a thin layer of condiments and no extras such as tomatoes or lettuce. If we're eating out and she orders a hamburger, I remove everything but the patty. I cut up the other contents so she can use a fork or spoon. I also cut the sandwiches into quarters because they're easier to handle. And the supersized monster burgers some places serve? Even I can't eat them.

I bought a sandwich maker that pinches the edges of the bread together, keeping the contents inside the pocket it creates. It's much more convenient.

Food that can be speared is preferable to food that has to be balanced on a fork or spoon. Potatoes are easier to eat than rice. Steamed vegetables are easier than pureed. And unfortunately for your budget, steak is better than meatloaf, unless your loved one has trouble swallowing. In that case, solid foods like steak can lodge in her throat and choke her. Use soft foods.

### Giving Medications

As any nurse can tell you, some people resist taking their medications. Some won't open their mouths, others will spit the tablets out. Still others will develop sneaky ways of making you think they've swallowed them only to dispose of them later—in some care homes, the potted plants are better medicated than some of the residents. If your loved one takes her medications without concern, you won't have a problem, but you still have to be diligent about making sure the tablets actually go down because sometimes she can inadvertently spit them up. So after she's finished, check the bottom of the water glass. Then check around her to see if a pill has fallen onto the chair or the bed or wherever she's sitting.

If she refuses to take her medications, you need to talk to your doctor to figure out how to administer them; not taking them isn't an option. One approach is to crush the pills up and put them in food or dissolve them in a drink she likes. This is fine for standard medications, but not for slow-release tablets such as Sinemet CR (CR means "controlled release"). Crushing these pills disables the gradual release of the medication. Your doctor may prescribe regular Sinemet but on a lower and more frequent dosage.

There have been two recent developments for administering Parkinson's medications. One is a skin patch that delivers a dopamine agonist called rotigotine; the other is an external pump that delivers levodopa/carbidopa directly into the intestine. The pump obviously has complexities of its own, but it's one way to ensure your loved one gets the medications she needs.

### Transferring

Over time, the disease will progress. Your loved one's mobility will decline and she'll have to make the transition to a cane, a walker, and ultimately a wheelchair. Wheelchairs are unfriendly to walls, and unfortunately some doors are too narrow for them. When Sandra was in a chair after her broken hip, I had to remove the doors from the bedroom and bathroom. Our guests had to rely on our discretion for their privacy. If her condition had been permanent, I would have installed a curtain-type door or, if I'd been feeling ambitious, a sliding door.

The day will come when you will have to help your loved one out of or into a chair or bed. Medical people call this "transferring." To transfer her, make sure your back is straight; use your legs to lift. You'll be doing a lot of it, and if you do it wrong, you'll be the person in need of help. Consult with an occupational therapist for advice on how to lift safely. One aid is a transfer belt, available from medical supply stores. It cinches around your loved one's waist so you can hold onto it as you lift her or help her walk. Some transfer belts are just strips of material with Velcro; others are more complex, with handles for you to grasp.

Without a transfer belt, there are two techniques for transferring. One is to hold your loved one by the hands or wrists, lean back, and pull her up toward you, standing her up. Now you can turn her so the chair or bed is behind her and ease her down. But this technique requires her participation. If she's not able to support herself, use the second technique. Facing her, slide your hands under her arms and hold onto her back. Bend your knees, hold her tight to you, and stand. Now you can swing her around to the bed or chair and sit her down.

If you're helping your loved one into bed and you need to shift her into the center, brace both your knees against the side of the mattress, place your hands underneath her lower back or buttocks and upper thighs, and slide her over. Bracing your knees protects your back.

I do have one advantage in helping her. She's lighter, smaller, and prettier than I am, so I'm able to lift her and support her with relative ease. If you're a woman and your loved one is your husband who is heavier than you are, talk to an occupational therapist about how to help him. There are useful devices such as tilting chairs, floor-to-ceiling poles, or patient lifts, and while some of them are expensive, they allow you to move your loved one from one place to another.

### Transferring into a Car

Transferring someone into a car can be difficult, particularly if the car is an SUV or van with a high seat. Here's how I transfer Sandra into our car—a sedan.

I open the car door and wheel her chair up to it, angled in toward the car. I've already swung the wheelchair footrests out of the way, so the chair is close to the door. Then I squat in front of her, put my arms under her armpits and around her back, and stand, lifting her. Then I pivot toward the car and ease her onto the seat. Sometimes, I let go of her with my left hand and push her hips into the car. Then I slide her onto the seat and swing her legs in. Finally, I ease my hands under her legs and slide her backward in the seat. Now that she's in place, I can buckle up the seatbelt.

Transferring her out of the car is much the same, but in reverse. I position the wheelchair at an angle to the open door with the footrests swung back. Then I undo her seatbelt and swing her legs out. I slide my arms under her armpits with my hands on her back, then I stand up, lifting her, and pivot toward the chair, seating her. Finally, I go behind the chair and pull her upright.

### Mobility

How do you help your loved one move around? Here's how I help Sandra. If she's having a better day, I walk beside her and hold one hand. If not, I stand in front of her and hold both hands. I've gotten really good at walking backward. If there's ever an Olympic event . . . However, according to one physiotherapist I saw, this is wrong: I should stand behind her and manipulate her hips to get her moving.

I have a big problem with this advice. If I do what the physiotherapist recommended and Sandra starts to fall, it's unlikely I can catch her. If I'm standing in front of her holding both her hands and she starts to fall, I can. In fact, it's not even correct to say I catch her. In most cases, I just stiffen up and let her catch herself.

If your loved one tries to walk but freezes and can't get started, here's a tip that worked for Sandra. Put your foot down in front of her at right angles to the direction she's trying to go and say, "Step over my foot." Most of the time, she will do so, which breaks the pattern and gets her moving. Another tactic that some people have recommended, although I never found it helpful with Sandra, is to march in place. Once your loved one is moving her feet up and down, she can start to move them forward.

### Falls

Your loved one will probably fall. Any emergency-services people will advise you to call 9-1-1 and have her taken to a hospital for evaluation. While this is the safest thing to do, there's a problem.

To protect your loved one's back and neck, the paramedics will place her on a rigid board and put a neck brace on her. Depending on how busy the emergency ward is, she could spend several hours before these are removed. This is brutal and the effect on Sandra is extreme: I found it was taking two or three days for her to recover from a visit to the hospital when, in most cases, there was nothing wrong. So we have become good at doing an assessment ourselves before we decide to call an ambulance.

When she falls, my first step is to check her demeanor. If she's annoyed, I ask her if she's okay, and if I get a clear response, I help her get up. Otherwise, I check for broken bones by rotating her arms and legs and pressing on her hips and chest. Broken bones are painful, so if there's no pain, she probably doesn't have one. I also check whether she suffered a concussion. And just in case her fall was from a stroke, I check for that as well. Here are some simple tests:

■ If your loved one is unconscious, breathing or not, call emergency services.

■ If she is bleeding from her mouth, nose, or ears, call emergency services.

- If she is conscious, ask her for her name and what happened. If she cannot respond or is confused, or her speech is unusually slurred, call emergency services.

- If she is nauseated, call emergency services.

- Ask her to smile. If she cannot, or the smile is unnaturally crooked, call emergency services.

- Ask her to stick out her tongue. If she cannot or the tongue comes out on one side, call emergency services.

- Shine a flashlight across her eyes. If the pupils don't constrict (shrink), call emergency services.

Otherwise, help her get up, help her to the bedroom, and let her lie down and rest.

It's also a good idea to keep a log of her falls, partly for her doctors to review and partly to head off legal charges. I talk more about that in the next chapter.

### Communicating

Communicating with someone with Parkinson's can be difficult because their voices tend to become softer and slurred. Complicating things is that one of the effects of Parkinson's is to impair decision-making. So if you want your loved one to make a choice, make it easy for her to answer. For example, instead of asking "What would you like for breakfast?" ask "Would you like toast or cereal?" You could even say, "I can make you toast or cereal. Would you like toast?" At times, Sandra tries to give an extended answer to a yes or no question, so imitating an aggressive television lawyer at trial, I'll say something like, "Would you like toast? Yes or no."

To help me hear her in a noisy place like a coffee shop, we got a portable speaker and a lapel microphone. I'd put the speaker on the table, clip the lapel microphone to Sandra's blouse, and plug it into the speaker. I found that it amplified her voice enough to make her words clearer. You can get these at most electronics stores. Get a single speaker, not a pair.

# Dealing with Dementia

The physical handicaps that Parkinson's imposes are bad enough, but to me, the symptoms of Parkinson's dementia are ghastly. Not only is your loved one losing the ability to feed or dress herself, but she begins to shift into a fantasy world of her own, one in which you are shut out. Sandra never moved there permanently: most of the time, she is lucid and as attached to the real world as anyone else. But occasionally, she is gone.

Her excursions into her new world take two forms. One is a sense of urgency: we have to do something and we have to do it now. Sometimes, it's clear what has to be done: we've lost the checks and we have to find them and put them in the bank. Of course, there are no checks. Other times, I cannot figure out what has to be done. All I know is that she is nearing panic, and the more I protest, the more anxious and insistent she becomes.

The second trip into her fantasy world is hallucinations. These aren't threatening, but they can be bothersome. We can't go out for coffee because we can't leave "him" alone. We have to be quiet or we'll wake "her" up.

When I first started dealing with these episodes, I believed it was my job to pull her back to the real world: to pry her out of her fantasyland. So I'd impose reality on her: there are no checks; there is no "him" or "her" to worry about. But the more I persevered, the more upset she became, which fueled my frustration, which increased her anxiety, which . . . well, you get the idea.

Nor was this a minor ripple in our lives. It was beginning to threaten my grip on my emotions. One evening, I became so frustrated I went into the backyard and screamed. Either my neighbors are deaf or uncaring or I don't scream loudly enough to trigger a visit from the cops.

Then one day, I read a book that someone in my Parkinson's caregivers support group had recommended: *Contented Dementia.*[*] At first I dismissed it. It describes a program developed in Britain for Alzheimer's Disease, and Sandra doesn't have Alzheimer's: her memory is better than mine. But while the techniques in the book didn't apply, the underlying principle began to make sense. The book points out that most relatives of Alzheimer's patients try to bring their loved ones back into the real world. Unfortunately, they can't go there, so anyone who gives care has to enter the patient's world. The book describes the problem:

---

* James.

> [People with dementia] are constantly reminded of their lack of value, as they find themselves cursing their inability to recall basic facts of their life and as others manifestly overrule them.

> But . . . things are only marginally better for the carer. . . . all too often, no one else seems to notice that you are busting a gut to try and keep them from falling apart.

> And yet it really does not need to be like this. . . . there is a simple method for dealing with . . . the daily behavioural problems, one which . . . [changes] the situation from one of personal hell to salvation.*

The suggestion that I get into Sandra's world resonated with me. Certainly, I was getting ragged trying to draw her back into mine. Perhaps the book had a point: rather than battling her, I needed to join her. The problem was I had no idea how to do it. So I consulted with one of Sandra's doctors, Andrew Howard, a neuropsychiatrist at the University of B.C. He described her episodes of urgency as similar to a waking dream or a strong feeling of déjà vu in which the person is convinced the images, like memories, are real even though, like a dream, they have no relation to one another or to reality. The approach he recommended was to assure her it was taken care of, whatever "it" was. As for hallucinations, he suggested acknowledging her feelings while not confirming them. He gave me a few scripts to help her.

So a couple of days later when she began panicking about the checks, I didn't insist there were no checks. I said, "What are you carrying on about, woman? I deposited them yesterday. It's all taken care of." She stopped, looked at me, and said, "You did?"

"Yes, I did. It's all taken care of." Instantly she relaxed and settled down. I was astonished, but to me the bigger test came a few days later when she was in a frenzy about something but I couldn't figure out what it was. So, taking a deep breath, I said, "Oh, yeah. I know what you're talking about. Yeah, you're right. We need to look after that. It's too late today, but I'll take care of it tomorrow. Okay?"

She looked at me, relaxed, and said, "Okay."

---

\* James, pages 95–96.

And I thought *Holy [expletive]*.

I've had similar results with her hallucinations. When she refers to "him," I'll follow the advice of her neuropsychiatrist, Dr. Howard, and say something like, "Yeah, it does kind of feel like someone's there, doesn't it?" Or I may say, "I don't see anyone, but it sure feels like there's someone there."

I won't pretend the problem has been solved. Her dementia is creative, always presenting more challenges. But with the attitude that my role is not to insist she return to reality but to make her comfortable in hers, my frustration level has plunged. And so has hers.

But this strategy did impose a hesitation I had to overcome. It required me to say things that weren't true. I hadn't put any checks in the bank and it didn't feel to me like anyone was there. *Contented Dementia* talks about this:

> That raises an immediate problem for many carers: . . . "How can I authentically agree to something I disagree with?" Penny's [Penny Garner, developer of the program] robust retort is that the carer must grow up and take responsibility. If they really want to protect their clients, . . . that means not imposing present-day reality unnecessarily.*

"Grow up" sounds a little harsh, but applied gently, I take it to mean "accept the responsibilities caregiving has imposed on you." And like pretending to young children that Santa Claus exists, the comfort of your loved one sometimes requires you to accept things you would normally challenge.

I also had another source of concern. Often, Sandra won't follow simple instructions. For example, when I put her in her wheelchair, I'd say, "Feet on the footpads." When she didn't comply, I'd repeat the instruction louder: "Put your feet on the footpads." On the third time, I'd add a few choice adjectives for emphasis. My goal was to demand she do this on the grounds that she should do as much for herself as possible. But to my frustration, it didn't work.

Dr. Howard explained there is a disconnection between the part of her brain that has the intent and the part that carries it out. She believes she is trying to put her feet on the footpad. The solution? If she doesn't do it herself, I do it for her. Simple, straightforward, and calming.

---

\* James, pages 110–111.

# 23

# The Structural Dimension

The structural dimension of caregiving is about creating an environment that supports you and your loved one and makes both your lives easier. What can you do in your home to help in her care? What can you do to reduce risks? What can you do to make traveling easier? Let's look at some things that might help.*

I'm not a therapist, physio or occupational, so I don't have professional qualifications to draw on. I can only describe what we did to ease Sandra's life. I guess I've had some success because when occupational therapists have done a home assessment, they haven't handed me a long list of things to upgrade. So I hope what I've learned will help you. There are many other devices or services, too many for this book, but the ones I've included here should give you an idea of where to start and what to look for. To conduct your own research, speak with your family doctor and neurologist. You'll find a wealth of information on the Internet. Look up "assistive devices" or "medical supply stores."

## Preparing Your Home

### Home Assessment

Most health services offer an in-home assessment of how you can modify your home. The people who do this are occupational therapists trained in spotting potential problems and who know what kinds of tools

---

\* For a thorough list, see Schwarz.

and technologies are available. Talk to your family doctor or neurologist to find out how to contact them.

Many devices such as staircase lifts, walk-in bathtubs, or overhead patient lifts are expensive, and you won't need them until your loved one's disease has progressed to the point where she needs total care. There are cheaper alternatives, which is good, because I'm cheap. Let's have a look.

### Flooring

The best choice for flooring is carpet. Hardwood or regular tile is poor, ceramic tile is the worst. Why? Drop a crystal glass onto each type of floor and imagine it's your loved one's hip or elbow.

Also, when a hard floor gets wet, it's slippery. That's not advisable for the surefooted, never mind Parkinson's patients or those who are helping them.

But there's another reason. Some people with Parkinson's tend to lean sideways or backward as they walk. If you're holding onto your loved one and she is leaning, her feet will slip. They'll slip less on carpet than on the other types of floor. If you don't want to change your hardwood floors, consider putting down area rugs with rubber backing. Don't use throw rugs unless you have a lot of medical insurance and really love visiting the hospital.

Since carpet is a poor choice for bathrooms and kitchens, in our bathroom we put rubber-backed bathmats on the floor and around the toilet. In the kitchen she's on her own, but since I do all the cooking, she's seldom there.

Carpet does have one disadvantage over hard flooring: it's more difficult to clean if there's a spill (although a glass of red wine spilled onto tile grouting can be a problem). Buy yourself a carpet steam cleaner. It will come in handy.

The only exception to carpet is if your loved one is confined to a wheelchair and can move herself around. It's easier to move a wheelchair on a hard floor than on carpet.

### Toilet

Getting onto or up from the toilet can be a problem. You can install a raised toilet seat, available at medical supply stores. Some of these just elevate the seat, but others have arms built in, which make it easier for the person to ease herself down or to get up. Some of them just slide onto the toilet so you can remove them when you have guests or you need to use the toilet yourself.

If your toilet is near a wall, you can install grab bars so that the person can lift herself up. Be careful of the toilet paper dispenser: it can become a makeshift handle, but normally it won't hold her weight.

Another option is a pole for the person to grasp. In our house, the vanity is in front of the toilet, so I attached a couple of metal rings to it and ran a thick wooden dowel vertically through them. I slit open a tennis ball and stuck it on the top of the dowel so that if Sandra slipped, she wouldn't give herself a tracheotomy. If you can't mount such a pole because of the layout of your bathroom, consider getting a floor-to-ceiling adjustable pole, available at some medical supply stores. If you get one, please consult the store or, even better, have someone install it for you. These poles are held in place by friction, and if they're not properly installed, they can slip loose. Some of them also have crossbars, which make it easier for your loved one to grasp. However, the pole is going to get in your way. Before you install one, think about whether the inconvenience and risk of having to work around it outweigh its advantages.

### Shower

Grab bars in the shower are mandatory. If you don't feel comfortable installing them, hire a handyman. If your shower wall is ceramic tile and you're confident or daring enough to try doing this yourself, use a ceramic drill bit. If you can't find a stud or it's in the wrong place, secure the screws with wall anchors. When you drill into ceramic tile, there are a couple of problems to be aware of: the tile doesn't take a pencil mark, and when you start to drill, the drill bit will wander and you won't get the hole exactly where you need it. Here's a hint: put a strip of duct tape over the spot. The tape will take the pencil mark and will also hold the drill bit in place until it bites into the tile.

A few words about wall anchors. There are several different types, each with its own purposes and strengths. If you install the wrong one, you're wasting your money and putting your loved one at risk. If you're not an expert in wall anchors, talk to someone at your local hardware store.

When the disease gets to the point where your loved one can't stand in the shower even with shower bars to grip, you can install a shower chair. There are two main kinds. The simplest is a chair that sits inside the tub or shower. It has drain holes, and some even have cutouts in the bottom for what the manufacturers coyly call "personal washing." Some chairs have backs, some have armrests, and some attach to the shower wall and can fold up when they're not being used.

The other type is a transfer bench. This chair sits partly in and partly out of the tub and is for people who can't step into it. The person sits on the outside part of the bench, then swings her legs over the sides of the tub and slides herself along the bench. Some transfer benches have a sliding seat.

The disadvantage of a transfer bench is that you can't keep the shower curtain inside the tub, so water will get out. A friend of mine placed the outside legs of the bench onto a boot tray, which caught most of the water. For the rest, he used towels.

Of course, for those with a larger budget, there are walk-in baths and even lifts to get the person into the tub.

Someone suggested that Sandra use a hand-held shower instead of a fixed shower head. But having to manipulate the shower as she was soaping herself was too much for her to handle, so we stuck with a fixed head until she could no longer shower herself at all. At that point, I got a hand-held head that I use when I'm showering her. I also got a "diverter valve," a unit that attaches to the shower outlet and can hold two shower heads: one fixed for me to use and one for the hand-held. You can also get a hand-held head with a bracket that keeps the head in place.

### Towel Racks

Towel racks are a hazard because someone who is unsteady will grab them for support. Since people tend to be heavier than towels, even wet ones, most racks can't take the weight, which means that not only does the rack break but the person ends up on the floor.

You could install grab bars and use them as towel racks, but you can also strengthen the racks you have, assuming they're not flimsy. Remove them and then re-attach them using wall anchors and heavier screws. If you can put the screws into studs, the rack will be stronger than if the screws just go through the drywall.

Depending on where the toilet paper dispenser is, you may also need to strengthen that. It can make a tempting handle for your loved one to grab as she gets up from the toilet.

A PARKINSON'S LIFE

### Staircases

If you have a staircase in your house, install a childproof door at the top and make sure it's always secure. If your loved one is mobile but gets confused, keep a latch on the door—one that's not easy to open.

Some staircases have banister railings that don't extend the full length of the stairs. If that's the case in your house, install railings that fill the gap. Even if you have to break the railing into two segments, a person walking up or down the stairs needs something to hang onto from top to bottom. Again, for money, you can install a lift chair that runs up the stairs and carries a person and a wheelchair. For your hallways, you can also install a horizontal railing, like a banister, for your loved one to hold onto.

### Doors

What if your loved one is in the bathroom or bedroom and falls against the door? If it opens inward, she'll be blocking it and you won't be able to get it open. If you force the door, you risk injuring her. You can solve this by reversing the direction the doors open so all inside doors open outward. This would be a substantial job requiring you to modify the doorframes. If you're not a handyman, talk to one.

Your loved one can inadvertently lock herself into a bedroom or bathroom and then not be able to unlock the door. Disable all inside door locks or get the kind that you can unlock from the outside. Otherwise, if she can't get out, you'll have no recourse but to kick in the door.

### Bedroom

If your loved one has difficulty getting out of bed, or conversely is at risk for falling out, you can get specialized beds. But they're expensive, so before you get there, there is a simple option: a portable bed rail. Imagine a long metal bar bent into a U-shape with a flat bottom. Now imagine it's lying on the floor and a 500-pound gorilla stands on it, grabs the bottom of the U, and pulls it up so it's vertical. There you have it. Slide the ends of the bar under the mattress and the U-shape comes up the side and forms a rail to help the person in and out of bed. This device is also portable; ours has been on numerous car trips and flights. You can find them on the Internet. Search for "portable bed rail."

If your loved one needs to visit the bathroom at night, install a commode beside the bed to avoid having to make the trek to the toilet. We installed two night lights. One is very low and doesn't disturb sleep; the other is brighter but motion-sensitive. When Sandra starts to get up, the brighter light comes on.

If you set up a commode, you may also have to install a toilet paper dispenser. The alternative is to use a box of facial tissues.

### Bed

You can simplify making the bed by using a duvet. Instead of having to tuck in a top sheet and blankets, simply fluff up the duvet and lay it down on the bed. You don't have to mess with a top sheet and there are no hospital corners to worry about. Sheet sets usually come with a fitted sheet and a flat sheet. With a duvet, you won't need a top sheet, so you can have a sewing store convert the flat sheet into a fitted sheet.

Make sure you have a standard-height bed. Avoid the ones with a high mattress; they're harder to get into. Also avoid the ones that are too low down, like a futon; they're harder to get out of. If you have a low bed, consider putting it on blocks or on a bed frame with a box spring.

If you use a duvet and want to convert a flat sheet into a fitted one, a high mattress won't work: many flat sheets are not wide enough to fit, which is another reason to stick with a standard mattress.

### Nighttime Accidents

If I were asked to come up with a slogan for caregiving, it would be, "Turn problems into nuisances." One of these problems is nighttime incontinence: bed-wetting or worse, especially if the mattress is damaged. Cleaning it can involve steam-cleaners, expense, and inconvenience. That's a problem you don't want to face.

Therefore, make sure you have a mattress cover, one that's waterproof or at least thick enough to absorb accidents. To provide extra insurance, get a couple of waterproof bed pads. These are large pads two or three feet wide, available at most pharmacies or medical supply stores. You put them under the bottom sheet (absorbent side up, please) so that if there's an accident, all you need to do is toss the sheet and pad into the washing machine and put on fresh ones. You have reduced a problem to a nuisance.

### Around the House

Rearrange the furniture so there are clear pathways. Parkinson's patients freeze in tight situations like doorways or that narrow space between the coffee table and the easy chair.

If your loved one is mobile, consider replacing your doorknobs with lever handles—they're easier to manage. Also, replace your light switches with large rocker switches. It's even better if you can get ones that have a light inside when they're off.

When you're going out, you may find that it's getting harder to help your loved one put on her coat because she's unstable when she holds onto a wall or door jamb. You can install a handle next to your coat closet for her to hang onto. You'll find these at the hardware store in the bathroom fixtures section as grab bars. Some of them are far more sleek and attractive than the typical steel bar. Ours actually looks like a slim wall telephone.

## Safety and Security

### Alarms

There will be times when your loved one needs help and you may not be within earshot. We installed a wireless doorbell, bought five buttons, and programmed them for the Westminster chimes (to distinguish them from our real doorbell). I installed two buttons in the bathroom—one by the toilet and one by the sink—using double-sided tape. The others are distributed around the house so that when Sandra needs help, she can press a button and I will hear the bell.

When Sandra can't get to a button, she calls for help. If I'm in my office downstairs, I can't hear her, so I installed a wireless baby monitor and put the speaker in my office. That way, if she calls out, I'll hear her—when I'm in my office. You can spend hundreds of dollars for a baby monitor, or you can get one that is perfectly fine at a discount retailer for about twenty-five dollars.

But what if your loved one needs help when you're not at home? You can register for a medical alert system. Your loved one will wear an alarm button, either as a pendant or a bracelet, which sends a signal to a controller attached to your phone line. The controller includes a loudspeaker and a microphone. When she presses the button, an attendant will come on the line and ask if she needs help. Some services claim that they can detect if the person has fallen; the system sends an alarm automatically. If you want to have one installed, search for "medical alert systems." If you search for "monitored alarm systems," you'll get systems that monitor for break-ins and fires.

The microphone is sensitive enough to pick up a call for help from a distance, and the attendant will call emergency services, even if your loved one can't speak. They will always call for help unless they're satisfied there are no problems. If Sandra bumps the button and sets off the alarm, I tell the attendant we're fine, but he often calls back a few minutes later to double-check.

I also arranged with the monitoring company for me to have my own alarm. One morning, I slipped and almost fell in the shower, and I realized that if I had a medical problem, it's doubtful Sandra could call for help. We could have ended up as one of those grisly stories on the evening news of people being found days after their neighbors reported a funny smell. So I also wear a bracelet on my wrist.

### Access

How do the emergency services people, fire or paramedics, get into your home? You could hide a key somewhere obvious, but that creates the risk that people you'd rather not have in your house could get in. I was also concerned that hiding a key might invalidate our insurance, so I called the insurance company and spoke to a very nice, if gullible, lady who said, "Oh, yes. You can hide a key. I keep mine . . ." Then she stopped. I considered asking her for her address.

Since I don't want to hide a key, I asked a paramedic how they'd get in if nobody answered the door. He said they'd breach it. "Breach" is emergency-speak for "smash it in." If you'd rather not have to replace or repair your front door, install a lockbox with a key to the house. You can get these at most locksmiths. They screw into the door frame and have a numeric pad on which you enter a code to open the box.

You get to set the code, but there's one caution. With inexpensive lockboxes, which are just as robust as their more pricey cousins, the sequence in which you enter the numbers on the code doesn't matter. I was planning to use "51342," my membership number in an organization I no longer belonged to, but the code "12345" would also open the box. So when you pick a code, pick one in which the numbers, when you put them in order, aren't consecutive.

You can also choose how many digits to have in your code. Five gives you the most combinations. Because the length of the code is up to you, that alone stymies potential burglars. Not only won't they know your code, they won't even know how long it is.

Once you've picked a code, give it to the alarm monitoring company to pass on to emergency services. Also, check whether your local ambulance, police, and fire departments have a service to register your code.

A lockbox is also convenient for home support services or hired care aides; they don't need to carry a key.

Finally, hang a small flashlight with your lockbox so anyone needing to enter can see the keypad when it's dark. Don't forget to test the flashlight from time to time.

### Notifications

I printed off Sandra's medication schedule, her allergies, and her DBS history along with a warning never to give her an MRI without a neurosurgeon's approval. These are in an envelope stuck behind the mirror in the bathroom. The envelope is labeled in large letters "Instructions to Paramedics for Sandra Hallows." The envelope also contains a small plastic bag with a day's medications. It's in the bathroom because that's where the paramedics normally go to look for the meds. If you prefer, you can attach one to your refrigerator with fridge magnets because the paramedics will also look there.

One of my big fears was of something happening to me while I was away from the house. If I were in an accident or had a medical emergency and was unable to talk—or worse—nobody would know about Sandra. I could carry an alert card, but I couldn't use her doctor's phone number or that of her home support case manager because they're only available during normal business hours. I needed someone who could be contacted at any time. So I arranged coverage with the local private nursing agency that we had used.

The letter I wrote to them with my requirements says, in part,

The purpose of these services is to ensure the safety of my wife, Sandra, in the event that I am in an emergency and unable to care for her. In such cases, Sandra could be alone and unaware of any problem.

I will carry a card marked "In case of emergency" instructing the authorities to contact your dispatch number, 555-555-5555, and inform the operator that I am in an emergency and to dispatch someone to care for my wife.

The detailed services that I would like you to provide are as follows:

1. Dispatch a care aide to my home (access details are in the original document I sent you). Instruct the care aide to
   a. Inform my wife of the nature of the emergency.
   b. Give any outstanding medications.
   c. Prepare and feed her any outstanding meals.
   d. Tend to any personal needs.
   e. If she needs medical care, call emergency services.
2. If the nature of my emergency is temporary—no more than one or two days—dispatch care aides to provide care for her during this period.
3. If the nature of my emergency is longer term or permanent, notify Sandra's case manager (details in the original document) and request a transfer to a respite home or care home. Also notify Sandra's family doctor.

I made up a wallet card about the size of a business card and had it laminated. The words on top of both sides of the card are in red.

| **In case of emergency** <br> **\* \* \* URGENT \* \* \*** <br> Call {nursing agency}24-hour <br> dispatch at **555-555-5555** <br> or **1-555-555-5555** <br> See reverse | **In case of emergency** <br> **\* \* \* URGENT \* \* \*** <br> Notify them that **Jolyon Hallows** <br> requires assistance for his wife. <br> Inform them of my condition. Request <br> assistance for **Sandra Hallows,** <br> **{Address}, Burnaby, B.C.** |
|---|---|

I also provided the agency with medical information about Sandra that includes the following:

- Personal information (Sandra's full name and date of birth).
- My contact information: home phone, cell phone, and email address.
- Her health care card number.
- Our family doctor's name and phone number.
- Her medical conditions.
- Her ambulatory status.
- Special medical instructions. For example, because Sandra has had DBS surgery, she is not to receive an MRI under any circumstances without a neurosurgeon's approval.
- Sandra's allergies.
- A list of her prosthetics (dentures, glasses, etc.).
- The code to the lockbox.
- The name of her case manager at the home care organization.
- Her list of medications and medication schedule.
- Where the medications are located.

I have to be careful if Sandra is going to be away from home, either at respite or at her day program. I don't want care aides to show up at our house and panic when she's not there, so I have to remember to let the agency know when she's not going to be home. Just in case, I put the phone numbers of both organizations in Sandra's chart so that if care aides arrive, they can follow up and make whatever arrangements need to be made.

### Medications

Since I dispense Sandra's medications, I keep them in their original bottles in the medicine cabinet. This presented a problem, as I sometimes didn't remember if I'd given her a particular dosing. I considered having our pharmacy put the medications in blister packs so I'd know if I'd given them. But I found them to be bulky and hard to store, particularly since we normally get three months' supply at a time. Our pharmacy doesn't charge for this service, but you should check with yours.

You should also chart when you give medications. I didn't for a long time, but I was getting tired of asking, "Did I give you your four o'clock meds?" So I made up a spreadsheet like the one below and keep it in the dining room. Each time I give Sandra her medications, I note the time. This doesn't help me remember to give them, but it does tell me when I forget and it allows me to say "Oh, bleep," instead of "Did I give you your meds?"

Each month, I just change the month on the spreadsheet and print off a new copy. I file the completed charts in a folder.

| Sandra Hallows Medication Chart | | | | | | | |
|---|---|---|---|---|---|---|---|
| January 2017 | | | | | | | |
| Date | 8:00 a.m. | 10:00 a.m. | 1:00 p.m. | 4:00 p.m. | 7:00 p.m. | Bed | Night |
| 1 | | | | | | | |
| 2 | | | | | | | |
| . . . | | | | | | | |
| 31 | | | | | | | |

Then I discovered an alternative system. I got a one-day pillbox with four compartments. Each evening after she's in bed, I pour Sandra's meds for the four times she gets them during the day. (She actually gets them six times, but I've never had a problem with the early morning or the bedtime meds.) That way, I now know whether I've given a particular dosing. I have the advantage of a blister pack without the inconvenience.

But sometimes I needed a blister pack. The first time I had the pharmacy prepare one, there was a problem: Sandra takes her medications six times a day plus a set if needed during the night. The standard blister pack assumes four doses a day, so the blisters are laid out in a grid of seven columns by four rows. The seven columns are for the days of the week, the four rows for the times the medications are to be given. One blister pack lasts most people a week. The pharmacy agreed to flip the rows and columns around. Now the seven columns are for the times of day and the four rows are for the days. One blister pack lasts four days.

This layout shows how it works.

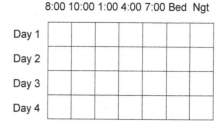

**A Typical Blister Pack Layout**

|      | Mon | Tue | Wed | Thu | Fri | Sat | Sun |
|------|-----|-----|-----|-----|-----|-----|-----|
| Morn |     |     |     |     |     |     |     |
| Noon |     |     |     |     |     |     |     |
| Eve  |     |     |     |     |     |     |     |
| Bed  |     |     |     |     |     |     |     |

**Sandra's Blister Pack Layout**

|       | 8:00 | 10:00 | 1:00 | 4:00 | 7:00 | Bed | Ngt |
|-------|------|-------|------|------|------|-----|-----|
| Day 1 |      |       |      |      |      |     |     |
| Day 2 |      |       |      |      |      |     |     |
| Day 3 |      |       |      |      |      |     |     |
| Day 4 |      |       |      |      |      |     |     |

I also bought a one-week pillbox, with the standard seven rows and four columns, and I relabeled them appropriately. This pillbox is in our living room for care aides to use whenever I'm going to be away for the day. Medications degrade over time, so whenever I refill a prescription, I replace the pills in the pillbox with fresh ones and use the old ones before I start the new prescription.

# Out and About

### Getting Out

We hadn't realized how much time we had spent window-shopping at the mall. Then Sandra's condition deteriorated until she couldn't walk any distance or stand still without holding on to something. The good news was that our budget benefited from the drop in impulse buying, but it was frustrating for her. Then we discovered that the mall lends wheelchairs. Since then, we've found that most malls and tourist attractions have wheelchairs to borrow.

We also discovered that some medical supply stores rent wheelchairs. So when the Winter Olympics were held in Vancouver, we rented one for the month so we could go downtown and enjoy the festivities.

For the longest time, we didn't buy one because every time I suggested it to Sandra, she grimaced and said no. I think she saw it as giving in. But the day finally came when she relented. Now we no longer need to rely on borrowed chairs.

### Wheelchairs and Ramps

When it was becoming clear that I would have to buy Sandra a wheelchair, I went into a medical supply store to look at what was available and get a feel for the cost. The salesman asked me questions about how we would use the chair, for how long, and where. When my answers were vague, he suggested I have someone assess her to recommend what she needed. Otherwise, we'd risk spending money on something that wouldn't work properly.

An occupational therapist did the assessment. She measured Sandra to determine the dimensions of the chair seat and the distance from the ground. She also asked us how we intended to use the chair. There's a vast difference in the type of chair for people who will use it occasionally and those who will spend most of their time in it. For one thing, people that spend a lot of time in a chair need a proper seat cushion to avoid getting sores, so there are cushions specially designed for this purpose. That cushion on your couch won't work.

The occupational therapist arranged for us to borrow a temporary chair from a local organization, and I was glad she did. The chair we got, although fitting Sandra's measurements, had handles that were too low; I had to bend over so much to push it that I was starting to feel like a troll (not that I knew where to find one). When I finally went to buy a chair, the height of its handles became one of my criteria. So before you spend money, try out a few chairs first. There will always be some glitch you hadn't thought of, and it's cheaper to find out on a loaner or short-term rental.

When you price out chairs, particularly if the occupational therapist has recommended a particular make, be ready for sticker shock. The frames of higher-end chairs can run around $2,000, a good seat cushion can cost $600, and an adjustable back cushion can run $800 to $900. Check out sources of second-hand chairs such as the classified ads or an online service. If you buy a second-hand chair, take it into a medical supply company to have it checked out and to fix any problems. You'll save a bundle.

If you need a ramp from your house and you're handy enough to try building one yourself, here are some tips. The standard slope of a ramp is 1:12, which means that for every inch of rise, you need twelve inches—a foot—of length. The average step is between six and seven inches high, so if you have six steps up to your house, that's a rise of about forty inches and you'll need a forty-foot ramp. If you have the space, fine. Otherwise, you'll have to get a ramp that has switchbacks or turns, which can make for exciting trips from your house but is far more complex to build than a straight run. When you calculate the length of the ramp, don't forget to factor in any slope of the ground. If it slopes up, you can use a shorter ramp.

If you don't have enough space for the length of ramp you'll need, you can make the ramp steeper. The 1:12 ratio is the standard, but if you're reasonably robust and your loved one is lighter, you can get away with a steeper slope; our ramp is twenty-four feet long for a rise of about thirty inches.

Building a basic ramp isn't hard. For ours, I made two 4 X 6 beams, twenty-four feet long. I used a set of 2 X 6 boards alternating six and twelve feet long and screwed them together. Each of my beams has two twelve-foot boards screwed to one twelve-footer and two six-footers.

The width of the ramp will depend upon the distance between the wheels of the chair. For most ramps, two feet is enough, but some chairs are wider. When you're measuring, remember that you'll need guides along the edges so the chair won't roll off, and you'll have to take into account the outer pushing rim of the wheels. For the floor of our ramp, I had the lumberyard cut two sheets of three-quarter-inch plywood lengthwise giving me four sheets of two feet by eight feet. I turned the beams on edge and attached the plywood to them with screws. Next, I screwed 1 X 4 boards along the edge so that the chair wouldn't roll off the side, and I cut a bunch of 1 X 2 boards into one foot lengths and screwed them to the plywood one foot apart to create steps. If you do this, remember that the steps can't go all the way across the ramp or your loved one will have a bumpy ride. Finally, I attached a couple of legs and a warning sign and stained the whole thing a deep red.

And that's it. Our ramp goes up to the second step below the landing because the thickness of the beams puts the top of the ramp in line with the landing. This means I have to muscle the wheelchair up the last step from the landing into the house, but that's cheaper than a trip to the gym. Now you may be about to say, "Hold on. You said that you'd built a platform on the landing." Good catch. I actually built two ramps: one when Sandra broke her hip and the one we have now. The new one doesn't have the platform.

The ramp doesn't have handrails because when I'm using it, both of my hands are on the wheelchair and I don't want Sandra to grab a railing.

If you build a ramp, don't do it without a power screwdriver. If you have a power drill, you can get screwdriver bits. Also, unless you welcome more frustration in your life, don't even think about using slotted screws; choose Phillips, or even better if you're in Canada, Robertson.

When we first used a wheelchair, I had problems getting it into the trunk of our car, not just because it was heavy but because it snagged on the mesh net I use to keep some semblance of order. So when we had the loaner chair, I figured out some complicated system with a sheet of plywood and a hinged flap that would fall over the top of the net. But as I was measuring the trunk to get ready to build it, I saw it had a large mat. So now I just pull the end of the mat over the net. It works fine.

### Handicapped Restrooms

Some places have separate restrooms for the disabled, but others just have handicapped stalls in their regular restrooms. I have helped Sandra in a women's restroom when there was no alternative; nobody has ever complained. Some shopping malls have family restrooms that can be used by both men and women, and they usually have a handicapped stall.

As Sandra's condition declined, she couldn't work the lock inside the restroom. I got so I could judge how well she was faring each day, and if I thought she couldn't handle it, I left the door unlocked and stood guard outside it, feeling like a centurion (although, again, I've never figured out where to find one).

I get angry at the able-bodied who use these restrooms. Apparently, some people use them for taking drugs, and I've seen couples emerge from them with embarrassed looks. I never fail to call them out and tell them they're taking advantage of the disabled. I've been told I shouldn't do this; I might encounter someone with an ice pick.* I guess antagonizing people is a risk, but I get annoyed at such thoughtless behavior.

### Handicapped Parking Permits

A handicapped parking permit will prove invaluable to you. You've seen these: they hang from a car's rearview mirror and bear a graphic of a person in a wheelchair. They allow the holder to park in designated handicapped

---

\*    I've never actually seen an ice pick despite numerous television pot-boilers where they're used as the murder weapon. I wouldn't even know where to get one. I'd make a lousy murderer.

parking spots. Your doctor can tell you whether your loved one qualifies and can requisition it or tell you where to get one.

There are two kinds of handicapped spots: close and wide. Close spots are near the entrance. Wide ones are extra wide to allow wheelchair access. Most spots are both close and wide.

The permit is either to be hung from your rearview mirror or placed on the dashboard when you park. I don't like hanging it permanently; it blocks my vision and it's also illegal to hang things from the mirror, although I doubt the law is ever enforced. Also, the mirror attachment in our car makes it awkward to hang the permit, so I stuck it to the sun visor with double-sided tape. Now all I have to do is flip down the visor whenever I park.

I have a personal plea. Don't use the permit to park in a handicapped spot if your loved one isn't with you. I know it's handy, particularly during busy periods at the mall, but you are affecting people who need the space more than you do.

On the other hand, don't be quick to judge someone who pulls into a handicapped spot and leaps out of the car without the slightest impediment. I've done that when I've dropped Sandra at the mall to get her hair done and then left on other errands. When I return, I park in a handicapped spot so she can easily get to the car, but of course when I do this, anyone watching would conclude that I'm alone and don't need the permit.

When you travel out of town, take the decal with you; it's recognized most places. Just don't forget it in a rental car. Getting a new one will be inconvenient.

### Traveling

We always keep a set of medications in the car in case I forget to bring them along when we're out and about. We also keep a couple of bottles of water in the cup holders for the back seats. There's also room for a box of facial tissues.

When you travel, hotels and motels can be a problem because most of them don't have facilities like grab bars in the shower. Some have handicapped rooms, but most don't. It pays to ask when you make your reservation or check in. Depending on your loved one's degree of mobility, you may need to insist on a ground-level room or stay in a hotel that has an elevator.

For showers, consider buying a glazier's lift: a device that glaziers use to heft heavy panes of glass. You can get one at most glass stores. It consists of two large suction cups connected by a bar. Unless the shower wall is rough or made of small tiles, you can attach it to the shower wall and use it as a grab bar. Ours is capable of holding two hundred pounds, far more than we need. I've also noticed that some bathroom stores now carry something similar, although they look flimsier.

You may find that the suction cups leave a rubber stain on the shower wall. It comes off with toothpaste.

When you travel by air, notify the airline of your loved one's needs. They'll do their best to accommodate you. You can arrange for a wheelchair at the airport and an attendant to whisk you through check-in and security and take you right to the gate. Some airlines let you borrow a wheelchair so you can wheel her yourself, which is handy unless you're loaded down with luggage.

If your loved one can't navigate the narrow aisle in the airplane, the staff will take her to her seat using a special wheelchair, although they will prefer to seat you near the front of the plane. Since this is probably also near a restroom, it's handy.

If this will be a long flight and it will be hard for her to get to the restroom, consider having her wear adult diapers that you can dispose of at the end of the trip.

Never put any medications in checked luggage. Never! Not a single pill! Here's a test: When can you put your medications in checked luggage? Answer: NEVER. Always carry them with you. If the airline loses your luggage, you'll still have them. Some people recommend just carrying a few days' medications and putting the rest in checked luggage. Don't. Even if your destination is within your country, you'll find it difficult, time-consuming, and expensive to replace them. If you're traveling outside the country, some places don't even have some of the medications you use.

When you plan for a trip, make a list of things you'll need including medications, nutritional supplements, and assistive devices. I've included a checklist in Appendix E: Traveling Checklist. It contains most of the normal items and some blank lines to add anything else you need. The safest way to make up such a list is to create it over a couple of weeks. Every time you use something, note it on the list. And don't forget to include things like false teeth and glasses, a list of medications, your doctor's phone number, and medical insurance cards. This list is also handy when you leave wherever you're staying. You can make sure that when you go, you have everything you came with.

### Travel Programs

There are numerous programs to help reduce your travel costs and to ease travel, both locally and beyond. For example, in Canada both major airlines allow attendants of the handicapped to travel domestically at no charge (although taxes and fees still apply). There are restrictions, but for those who qualify, the savings can be substantial. Many airlines will also waive the baggage fee for assistive devices—wheelchairs, walkers, or specialized equipment.

Locally, the transit authority offers several programs. One allows attendants to travel on public transit for free. Another provides taxi vouchers for half-price. Check with your local transit system to find out how they can help.

Other transit services have similar programs. Locally, B.C. Ferries, the company that services the coastal communities, allows residents to apply for a program that allows the disabled and their attendants to travel at a reduced rate.

Many of these programs require a handicapped person to apply for a card and to provide a doctor's approval, and they'll vary across states and provinces. But it's worth doing some digging to find out what's available.

## Community Resources

There are a large number of resources and programs in most communities to help those with chronic diseases like Parkinson's. Unfortunately, since they cost the system money, most people who work in the health care field won't tell you about them unless you ask specifically. Because of this, and because as the population ages the number of programs grows beyond what most people can grasp, there is an emerging group of advisors whose job is to tell you about the programs that are available and for which you might qualify. I've met several people whose loved ones have Parkinson's who, upon hearing of a program, said, "I wish I'd known about that." I've said it myself.

Support groups are excellent sources of information. Seek out a caregiver support group. You'll find people who have been through what you're going through and know about programs and services that might help.

If you live in a larger town, there may be adult day programs where you can drop your loved one off in the morning and pick her up in the afternoon. They'll feed her and give her her medications, but most important they offer a social atmosphere in which she can interact with others and get some stimulation beyond the walls of her home. Also, having her go there gives you time to yourself.

Some cities have community recreation centers that offer exercise programs for the elderly or disabled. Some of these focus on seated exercises, which reduce the risk of falls. Another benefit, should you see it that way, is that while your loved one is in the program, you can work out in the center's gym (as opposed to devouring a sugar-filled pastry in the coffee shop).

You can also check with a local Parkinson's office. These are usually affiliated with or run by national organizations and will have information on what's available in your area, including support groups for Parkinson's patients.

### Care Aides

Care aides are trained and licensed to provide home care. Their services may be available from government programs or from private nursing agencies. Government programs typically restrict the number of hours they can give and the services they can offer, while private agencies will be more flexible. For example, the health authority that covers Burnaby won't allow their care aides to give medications, regardless of how they're packaged. They can't even remind patients that it's time to take their medications. But the private agencies are under no such restrictions; their care aides will even give the medications that I keep in the labeled pillbox.

They also differ in what they'll do. The care aides from the health authority are cheerful and friendly, but they will do little other than give Sandra something to eat or drink or help her in or out of bed or to the bathroom. They're not required to clean dishes or wipe the table after she's eaten, although some do. The private care aides, on the other hand, are extremely helpful. We use a private nursing agency because the manager has been more than supportive and their care aides seem to have a low threshold for boredom. One even did the ironing while I was away one evening, then she folded the clothes and put them away—in the right place. I was impressed. Another reorganized our refrigerator. It looked far neater than it had been, but there was a downside: it took me a week to find the mustard.

Be aware that care aides, private or government, will not pick your loved one up if she falls. There are three reasons. First, most of them aren't strong enough and most workers' compensation organizations limit the weight that any worker is allowed to lift. Second, they aren't trained to assess whether she needs medical care. Third, if they try to help her and she slips, they could make the situation worse and open themselves up to injury and even legal action. So if your loved one falls, they'll call emergency services and make her comfortable while they wait.

You can hire care aides privately. If you do this, you are their employer, responsible for paying them and handling standard employment responsibilities such as tax deductions and payment for vacation time and statutory holidays. This sounds complicated, but an accountant can manage the paperwork for you. And there are advantages: you can specify what services you want the care aides to carry out, such as helping your loved one with exercises designed for people with specific needs. You can also specify the number of hours of coverage you need, and if you have room in your house, you can actually hire a care aide to live in.

If you choose this route, get some advice from health care employment agencies. Hiring people full-time can be expensive, and by law most employees can't be made to work more than a certain number of hours per week. If you need full-time coverage, you'll need several care aides. Some health authorities, recognizing that even full-time care coverage is less expensive for them than residential care, will subsidize the cost of care aides.

### Respite

There will be times that you won't be at home for several days. You may be on a business trip, or you could just need a well-deserved break. If you don't have caregivers at your home full-time, you can place your loved one in a respite home. This is usually a standard nursing care home that has some beds available on a short-term basis, but some care homes have a section set aside specifically for respite. Sandra stays in the Respite Hotel, a facility in a care home called Queen's Park Hospital. To say that she enjoys going there would be a stretch, but she doesn't mind it and the staff are always supportive and helpful.

The respite staff will need the full set of information about your loved one, including the medication schedule and her specific needs. Unless your loved one has demands that exceed normal care, the facility will be fully equipped to handle her. And what's "normal care"? They'll dress your loved one, feed her, help her with mobility, and assist in personal hygiene, and if there's an emergency, they'll either respond with their own internal resources or arrange transport to a hospital. Most respite homes also allow their guests to participate in the social activities they offer their regular residents, and many have facilities such as hairdressers or manicurists.

One piece of advice: if you place your loved one in respite to give yourself a few days' rest, don't visit her. I made that mistake the first time I stayed in town while Sandra went into respite. I'd visit her in the afternoon and take her out for coffee, but when I returned her to the care home, she'd want to come home with me. She couldn't understand why she had to go back. At times she was in tears. It was a struggle every day, and I felt like a jerk for leaving her there only because I needed a break.

So now when I put her in respite, I make up some story about having to go out of town. I feel bad about lying to her, but not as bad as I'd feel visiting her and not taking her home. And not as bad as I'd feel without having some relief.

But there's another consideration. I suspect Sandra's reaction was not just about wanting to come home but about fearing she would be abandoned. So now whenever I leave her in respite, I call her every day, usually in the morning, and I always say something like, "I'll be back next Sunday," or "I'll see you in three days." I believe my calls reassure her I'm coming back and she won't be stuck there permanently.

## Handling Legal Issues

### Legal Defense

If your loved one is prone to falling, you face a legal risk. A doctor who finds bruises or abrasions and who suspects abuse may report his or her concerns to the police. In some jurisdictions, doctors are required by law to do so. If that happens, you will be caught in a legal quagmire. I'm not a lawyer, but a casual glance at events tells me that for some charges, legal protections such as the presumption of innocence are weak or even nonexistent. Police and judges don't appear to have much sympathy for potential abusers, even if the evidence of abuse isn't clear.

Someone suggested to me that I keep a log of Sandra's falls. The log contains the following information:

- The date and time that she fell. If I'm not sure of the time, I approximate it.

- How I found her. Did I hear her fall or call out? Did I come home and find her on the floor? Did someone else find her? Was her monitored alarm triggered?

- What I did. What assessment did I perform? Did I call emergency services?

- Where she fell. Be specific. "In the bedroom" is not enough. Where in the bedroom did she fall?

- Difficulties in helping her. Was she jammed into a tight spot? Did she fall against a door and was she blocking it shut?

- Bruises and abrasions. Where were they and what was their extent?

- Any other relevant comments.

This log establishes a history of falls and bruises. It also describes where her bruises are and how old they are so that medical staff can compare what they find with your log. Keeping this log provides you with a defense against charges of abuse, and it can also be useful for your doctor in determining if there are any emerging patterns in her symptoms.

### Legal Representation

Being a caregiver of someone who is, or will become, incapable of handling her affairs means you'll need to look after the medical and financial aspects of her life. Doing that legally means having some form of legal representation such as a power of attorney. Because laws vary in different countries and in different provinces and states, there's no one approach that works for everyone, so you'll need to consult with a lawyer to determine what you need to put in place. You should also consult with medical or care professionals such as a case manager because some jurisdictions have simplified forms of representation that don't require expensive legal services. With Sandra, for example, I was able to use a "Representation Agreement" that allows her to consent to my making decisions for her.

When you explore representation, there are some factors to consider. First, do you need to handle her medical decisions, her financial decisions, or both? Some powers of attorney deal only with the financial aspects.

Second, does she need representation now or is she assigning it for some future time when she will?

Third, is she mentally capable of making the decision to assign you as her representative? If not, you will have to prove she needs representation.

Fourth, if she is capable, does she refuse to name you or anyone else as a representative? If so, and assuming she is not capable of managing her affairs, there are legal processes in place to force representation, but they are onerous and probably expensive. They are, after all, designed to protect people from having others take over their lives.

### Permanent Care Homes

At some point, your loved one will probably need to go into a care home. Long before that happens, you need to do some research. How can you select the home that's best for you both? How can you make sure that, if you also need care, you can both go to the same home so you and your loved one can remain together? What are the procedures for getting admitted? Do you need to document the level of care your loved one will receive? What's the difference between private and government-run homes? How much will it cost?

Most communities have resources to help you set up whatever is necessary so when you finally need to place her into a care home, you're not overwhelmed by the pressure to make decisions about things you don't understand. Your doctor or case manager can direct you to resources and sources of information.

### Insurance

When your loved one is diagnosed, study any medical insurance policies you have. What do they exclude? Will they cover her medications? Surgery? Treatments such as physiotherapy? You may find, for example, that your policy covers physiotherapy but not exercise therapy. Can you get the therapist to classify his or her work such that it's covered?

It's hard to buy insurance after your loved one is diagnosed, but you might check with your insurer to find out if you can extend an existing policy, particularly if it's a group policy such as one provided by an employer.

If a doctor recommends an expensive procedure, check your policy and double-check with your insurance agent. You don't want to get hit with a bill for something you had assumed was covered.

## Evaluations

How can you know if a doctor is competent or helpful? How do you determine whether a new treatment is useful? How do you figure out whether that website that offers relief is authentic or just a scam? In other words, how can you evaluate what's available? Let's have a look.

### Doctors

Your loved one's care hinges on the quality of the doctors that treat her. If you spend as much time evaluating a doctor as you would a new big-screen TV, you'll be more satisfied with the results. There are two things to consider: logistics and relationship. If you have just moved to the area and don't have a family doctor, check with friends or co-workers to get a recommendation or visit evaluation websites such as Rate MDs*. But be skeptical. Internet reviews, whether of doctors or anything else, aren't always trustworthy. We once booked a hotel in New York that had several nasty comments. We found that none of them applied to our visit.

To help you evaluate a doctor, here's a set of questions. They're in two groups: logistics questions and relationship questions.

### Logistics

- Does the doctor accept your medical plan? If not, what additional costs will you have to incur?
- How easy is it to get to the doctor's office? Do you have to climb stairs? Is there an elevator?
- Is parking nearby and easily accessible?
- How quickly can you see the doctor? What's the average waiting time?
- Does the doctor have privileges at the hospital of your choice?

---

\*    http://www.ratemds.com/

## Relationship

- Is there anything about the doctor that could cause relationship problems? This might seem politically incorrect, but if a patient would be uncomfortable with a doctor because of sex or age or ethnicity, then it's okay to find one with whom he or she can discuss personal and sensitive issues.

- Do you feel rushed, as if the doctor wants to get on to the next patient or afternoon golf game?

- Does the doctor take the time to ask pertinent questions?

- Does he or she listen to the answers?

- Does the doctor answer your questions fully and patiently?

- Does the doctor inform you of new treatments or services without your having to prompt him or her? Be wary of a doctor who only recommends treatments you suggest.

- Does the doctor explain things in a manner you can understand?

- Does the doctor treat you and your loved one with respect?

Don't confuse being nice with being competent. If I had to choose, I'd pick competence; being nice is what friends are for. If you're dissatisfied after you come away from a visit with a doctor (and appreciate that even good doctors can have bad days), particularly if your reaction extends to more than one visit, look for another doctor. Will you hurt his or her feelings? Perhaps, but you are your loved one's caregiver, not the doctor's. If you have concerns about a specialist, call the doctor who referred you, register your dissatisfaction, and ask for a referral to a different specialist. For example, Dr. Frame once referred me to an ear-nose-and-throat specialist because I was having problems with my ears. The specialist diagnosed me with tinnitus, but I wasn't satisfied that he had been thorough, and when I went online to learn about the condition, the symptoms weren't at all what I had. When I reported this to Dr. Frame, his opinion confirmed what my research showed: whatever the problem was, it wasn't tinnitus. He referred me to another specialist.

Take some time to learn about the condition and watch out for comments or diagnoses that don't match what you've learned. Even doctors can rush and make mistakes. You may have heard the old joke: what do you call a doctor who graduated dead last in his class? Doctor.

## Medications

Medications will become part of your life. Your loved one's doctors will prescribe things you won't even be able to pronounce. How can you begin to make sense of them, and more importantly, how can you evaluate them?

Drugs have different actions and side effects in different people. For example, Sandra could not tolerate the side effects of alendronate for her osteoporosis, but hundreds of thousands of other people use it without a problem. So when you hear horror stories about a drug, don't assume the same thing is going to happen to you or your loved one. When Sandra was prescribed a dopamine agonist called pramipexole, what I found was scary: one of the side effects was a reduction of inhibitions leading to excessive gambling, shopping, and even sex. Fortunately, Sandra had none of these nasty side effects, and the medication worked wonders for her. On the other hand, please don't think that just because a medication is available, your loved will be able to tolerate it and it will work. Sandra has tried several without any benefit, and some have made things worse.

Ignore websites and blog comments typical of the denizens who lurk in the basement of the Internet. Anyone who disparages a drug because it didn't help him or someone he knows or someone he heard about is a vicious busybody. Some people have suggested that these comments serve a purpose by highlighting adverse side effects of a medication. I disagree. They only cause panic or worse, steer people away from treatments that can help. Teaching about the side effects is the role of your doctor and your pharmacist, not some anonymous twit (or tweet).

Here are some questions to ask when your doctor recommends a new medication:

- What are the major side effects?
- What percentage of people get each one?
- Are the side effects permanent or will they disappear if the medication stops?
- What are the first symptoms of a side-effect problem?
- What is the absolute minimum dose to start with, and how often and by how much should the dose be increased to reach the optimum level?

Complicating the matter, doctors will sometimes prescribe a medication for "off-label use." What does that mean? Consider a medication that was approved to treat, say, Alzheimer's disease. Its documentation will describe the condition for which it is to be prescribed (Alzheimer's), how it is to be administered (tablet, liquid, injection, patch), and its dosage. But a doctor can prescribe it for a completely different condition if he or she believes it might be effective. This is legal—although it's not legal for the manufacturer to say it can be used for this other condition.

An example is the gabapentin Dr. Dian prescribed for Sandra. Gabapentin is used to treat epilepsy, but because one of its side effects is drowsiness, Dr. Dian thought it might give her a deeper sleep so she wouldn't have to get up so often at night. Why didn't he just recommend a sleeping pill? I don't know. I deferred to his judgment at least long enough to try it. And it worked for her.

Once your loved one starts a new medication, monitor for the side effects, particularly the more serious ones. Sometimes, this will require blood tests. For example, if your loved one is prescribed tolcapone, she should also be given a requisition for frequent liver function tests. When you fill a new prescription, your pharmacist will discuss how the medication is to be taken—with or without food, how often during the day—and will also give you information on the medication and its side effects. If your loved one experiences problems that would require hospitalization or at least a visit to the doctor, follow the instructions to the letter. It's true that some medications are forgiving: miss a dose and it won't have much effect. But others aren't, and you're (probably) not qualified to tell which is which. So don't mess with the medications and don't be cavalier about any side effects.

### Pharmacists

Pharmacists are underrated. Enroll them in helping you. If you think your doctor has been offhand in describing the side effects of a prescription or the interactions with other medications, talk to your pharmacist. He or she won't be able to change the prescription, but you will be armed with professional information when you go back to your doctor (or another one). Pharmacists will let you know how to take medications (time of day, with or without food, the effects of alcohol), and they'll also get to know your loved one's medications and needs. Above all, they are not order-takers. They will warn you if a new medication interacts with other drugs she's taking, and if your prescription changes, they will double-check with you to make sure you know.

Our pharmacy will package Sandra's medications in blister packs for just a few days, and they even agreed to modify the packs for her medication schedule. They also provide excellent service. When a care aide who was looking after Sandra called them to report that a pill was missing from one of the blisters, they immediately sent over an assistant with a replacement pill—only to discover that the original pill was there, stuck to the side of the blister.

## Products

The Internet is clogged with websites extolling new products that organizations have developed for people in need. When you're dragged down by the demands of caregiving and willing to try almost anything, it's easy to succumb to a sales pitch. But because you can spend a lot of money chasing phantoms, you need to be skeptical. I am not attacking care products, nor am I critical of new ones; we use several, and I respect the skill that goes into developing them. But there are two issues. The first is whether the product would work for you and your loved one. The second is whether the product works at all. Here's a sample of the kinds of things that can seem compelling.

### New Treatments

Suppose you visit a website offering stem cell therapies or gene therapies or special physiotherapies for people in need. How do you evaluate it? Here's the first test: are these therapies specifically for Parkinson's? There have been some successes in stem cell or gene therapy for some conditions, so it's easy to proclaim from these results that the therapies are helpful. But if a website or brochure doesn't mention Parkinson's or has the disease embedded in a long list of other conditions, forget it. If even the sellers of the therapy don't believe it works on the disease, why would you? And remember, a treatment that cures everything or almost everything is called a "panacea." In reality, the only thing it will treat is the seller's bank account.

But what if the treatment is focused on Parkinson's? First, get your doctor's opinion. He may not have heard of it, but that doesn't necessarily disqualify it. If you want to pursue it, contact the provider and ask for some references. If they refuse because of medical confidentiality, forget about them. Companies that sell therapies that work are happy to give references, and their satisfied customers are usually more than willing to tell you just how wonderful the treatment was and how it changed their lives.

When you check references, make sure you get names of some people who are local and with whom you can meet. Before Sandra consented to DBS surgery, we met with one of Dr. Honey's patients, who showed us his system, how it worked, and what he looked like when it was turned off. His comments went a long way to easing Sandra's concerns.

When you check references, be careful: some marketers will provide you with fictitious names or those of confederates. You can get around this by getting your doctor to contact a reference's doctors for an opinion. If a reference won't give you the name of his or her doctor, it's not a reference you can trust.

Don't contact a reference's doctor yourself. In the first place, he or she won't (and certainly shouldn't) be willing to discuss another patient's medical status. In the second place, the doctor could also be a confederate. Does this sound paranoid? Remember that bogus therapies are a huge business with large fees and expensive products and services. To a con artist, they're worth some effort to create deception. Paranoia is better than bankruptcy.

Here's a set of questions to determine whether to proceed with a treatment you've heard about but your doctor hasn't. If you answer no to any of them, forget about this treatment.

- Does the company providing the treatment give you references?
- Are some of the references local (at best, they'll be in your city, but at least they need to be in your country) and are you able to contact them personally?
- Are the references willing to give you the names of their doctors?
- Are the references' doctors registered with the appropriate medical association? (You could probably confirm this yourself, but it may be easier for your doctor to do so.)
- Can your doctor confirm that the references' doctors know of this treatment and will state that it was effective for their patients?

When all of these conditions are true, then and only then should you consider proceeding.

## Devices

Before you shell out a lot of money for some great new device or aid, see if you can assess it inexpensively. For example, I learned of a headband that superimposed a checkerboard pattern on the ground ahead of the wearer. When people with Parkinson's freeze, one way to help is to give them a pattern they can step over, similar to the "step over my foot" technique I mentioned earlier. Some sources recommend laying colored tape on the floor to create a grid to help people walk. This device is based on that concept.

The system sounded intriguing, but it cost over $1,000. Was there a way to test the idea with Sandra before we spent the money? Well, I needed a checkerboard pattern, so I went to a local hardware store and got them to cut a sheet of plywood in half lengthwise, giving me a strip two feet by eight feet. Then I got some self-adhesive, square-foot, cheap black and white floor tiles and stuck them in a checkerboard pattern onto one side of the plywood. Finally, I laid the plywood tile-side down and had Sandra walk along it several times while I timed her. Then I turned it over and had her walk over the tiles. Her average time was slower when she walked on the tiles. The bad news was that the device probably wouldn't have worked for her. The good news was that we'd just saved some money. But I repeat: just because it didn't work for her doesn't mean it won't work for your loved one.

We heard about a cane with a spring-loaded bar at the bottom. When the person using it freezes, he or she can flip a lever on the cane handle, the bar will drop down, and the person can step over it to get going. There's an up-to-date version that projects a laser line on the floor in front of the user. Of course, for this to work, the person has to be able to use a cane, so I got a regular cane for Sandra and had her try it before we bought the fancy one. It was a flop. She never mastered a normal cane, so the new device would have been useless to her.

# 24

# The Emotional Dimension

Caregiving is an emotional pit. It's bad enough for doctors and nurses and social workers and other professionals who come to care for the people they help and who grieve when those people decline. For us as caregivers it's far worse. In part, that's because we haven't learned—as the professionals have—how to distance ourselves from those we're caring for, and in part it's because we don't want to: we're dealing with people we love. Learning how to handle emotions, with or without therapy, is essential.

I have to admit I'm reluctant to discuss this topic. In the first place, I'm not a therapist, so I'm not at all qualified to advise anyone else. In the second place, we all deal with problems differently; my solution may not work for you. By the way, you may have noticed I seem to be spending a lot of time telling you what I'm not. But I'll bet you're none of these things either. That's not an accusation, it's a recognition that caregiving does not confine itself to those who are prepared. And it's an invitation: if I can handle this, you can too.

And I have to discuss it because the emotional aspect of caregiving is so critical that I can't ignore it. So in the next few sections, I'll describe what we did. This isn't strong advice like reinforcing towel racks. It's more an outline of the kinds of issues that you may face and some ideas on how I handled them. Please use them or ignore them as you see fit.

## Traditions

Like all married couples, Sandra and I have our traditions, especially around festive occasions. For example, at Christmas we decorate a tree and prepare Christmas stockings—actually gift bags—of small items: some useful, some whimsical, some fattening. But as Sandra's health has declined, she can't participate in any of this, so I was faced with a decision: to carry on the traditions or, recognizing that they're a lot of work, to give them up.

I decided to carry on. Yes, Sandra can't help decorate the tree, but even today, once the baubles are in place, she looks at it and says, "This is the most beautiful tree we've ever had." That sentence is a tradition.

I still prepare the stockings because she's always delighted to go through them. And I buy and wrap a gift from her to me because she wants me to have something under the tree. The good news is that it's always something I want, and one of us is always surprised.

She doesn't wear jewelry much anymore, but I still get her some because her eyes light up when she sees it.

I maintain these traditions because they give her joy. But I also maintain them because to do otherwise would be to give up: to acknowledge that the life we made together was over.

## Relationships with Others

You will need to tell your friends and family that your loved one has been diagnosed with Parkinson's. When is that and how do you tell them?

I don't remember when we told others. I do know that we told them in person except for a few, like my sister, Christine, who lived too far away for us to easily visit. We told her and a few others over the phone.

How did we tell them? Directly. "We have some bad news. Sandra has been diagnosed with Parkinson's disease." Most of them won't know what that means, and their reactions will vary. Some will want information. What is Parkinson's? Is it curable? Is it contagious? Others will offer support and sympathy. For those who want information, give it. For those who just want to support you, let them.

And there will be others who will tell you they're sorry, then they'll disappear. You'll never hear from them again. If you or your loved one calls them to suggest getting together, they'll tell you they'd love to but they just aren't available right now and they'll call you later. They never will. Bid them good-bye and give your affection to those who remain.

## Patience

People with Parkinson's move slowly. That means that the practice of rushing out of the house at the last minute isn't going to work anymore. Everything will take longer, including putting on her coat, making sure she has her purse and glasses, walking to the door, getting to the car, buckling in. And of course before you leave, she will want to visit the bathroom. If you have to be driving away from your home by a specific time for an appointment, you must start to get ready to leave at least fifteen minutes before you plan to put your car in gear.

## Changes in Your Relationship

One of the more devastating aspects of being a caregiver is that your relationship with your loved one changes. She is no longer a life partner, participating equally in the decisions you as a couple make, and she can no longer join you in the activities you once shared. She is now a patient, requiring you to make the decisions for her. From large decisions such as where to vacation or how to invest, to small decisions such as which movie to see or which restaurant to visit, to minuscule decisions such as which clothes to wear or which television program to watch, you are now the decision-maker. Furthermore, as your loved one's disease progresses, the scope of your decisions will narrow down. There will come a time when the choice of vacation spots is irrelevant because she can't travel; when the choice of restaurants doesn't matter because she can't eat out.

This change in your relationship is perhaps one of the hardest things to deal with because, like it or not, you now have a patient to care for, not just a spouse to love.

These changes lead to another emotional response: grief. We normally associate grief with the death of a loved one, but grief is about loss. You are losing a relationship and it hurts. Furthermore, the grief won't be the soul-wrenching pain of the death of someone close to you, an ache that resolves with time. It will be gradual and relentless. It may manifest itself as depression or anger or an unusual emotional response to events that are unrelated to you. Let me give an example. I was watching a news report of a funeral for some police officers who had been killed on duty. I had no connection to this story: I didn't know the officers, and the place where they were killed was on the other side of the country. In the past, I would have allowed myself a moment to reflect on the senselessness of it all, then moved on. But watching the funeral, my eyes started to water and I realized I was crying. I've since learned that events I would formerly have shrugged off have become far more profound. I attribute this to a form of grief. What have I done about it? So far nothing, because it hasn't become debilitating or even problematic. It's just a change in my psychology that may or may not need some attention in the future. For now, it's enough for me to be aware of its effects so I recognize them and can attribute them to something instead of wondering if my grip on reality is loosening.

## Taking Care of Yourself

Those who deal with caregivers are adamant about one thing: look after yourself. If you collapse, you won't do your loved one any good, and both of you will end up needing care.

But what does it mean to look after yourself? Here's how I handled it. In offering this, I'm not prescribing what you should do, I'm just giving you some examples. You'll find your own as long as you look.

I have an online business. This allows me to work at home, which is both a blessing and a curse. It's a blessing because I'm always there when Sandra needs me. It's a curse because I'm always there when Sandra needs me. But it gives me an outlet: something other than Parkinson's to focus on. If you have a job, whether in your home or outside, that's your outlet. Whatever your personal situation, you will need something other than your loved one and her condition to be a target for your attention.

In the evening after Sandra has gone to bed, I take about an hour to read a newspaper or a book or to play Sudoku, one of my fun recreations. Whatever I do, it transports me away from being a caregiver.

Sometimes in the afternoon if Sandra lies down for a nap, I'll tell her I have a couple of errands to run and will be back shortly. Then I go to a coffee shop and just sit and read a newspaper in the winter or admire the passing throngs of scantily clad young women in the summer. (Someone once accused me of being a dirty old man. I replied that I'm working on it.)

I joined a Parkinson's caregiver support group that meets once a month. Listening to others and their struggles doesn't make mine any easier, but it does help me understand that what's happening to Sandra and me is not unique. Not only do others give support and a sympathetic hearing, they're also a valuable source of information about services I hadn't heard of, and they're full of useful tips. For a long time, I was reluctant to join; I didn't think I needed to hear others' depressing stories. But I discovered that these groups aren't labeled "support" for nothing. We listen to one another, we empathize, and we help. I've grown close to the people in my group, and I look forward to our monthly meetings.

Occasionally, I put Sandra into respite and take a few days for myself. But it's hard for me to leave her alone because I miss her. As far as she is concerned, I'm out of town at a conference at an airport hotel. I started using this rationale because several years ago, Sandra came with me to a conference at an airport hotel so she could do some sightseeing while I was in the sessions. But the hotel was in an industrial area with nothing around it but warehouses and one chain restaurant. The next time I had a conference there and asked her if she wanted to come with me, she just said, "You go." Since then, when I need some respite time, I tell her that's where I'm going. She doesn't at all mind staying home. Yes, it's sneaky, but I get a break and she doesn't feel abandoned.

Of course, one of the downsides is that I can't even take pictures and show them to her or talk about what I did. But when I visited my brother and lamented that I couldn't show Sandra the family pictures I'd just taken, he said, "Do you mean the pictures I just emailed you?" He's as devious as I am. Must be genetic.

### Setting Limits and Guidelines

I attended a workshop for caregivers where the speaker urged us to set limits and guidelines and to clarify what we won't do. When I first heard that advice, I figured it came from someone who has never had to care for anyone else, because within my physical abilities, there is nothing I won't do if Sandra needs it. For example, you may insist that you could never clean your loved one after a bowel movement. But when the day comes that that's the only way to keep her clean, you'll have to abandon that limit or you can no longer fulfill your role as a caregiver. Caregiving requires numerous unpleasant activities, including providing personal hygiene, so saying in advance that you'd never do them is futile. True, things such as giving a sponge bath can be done by care aides, but these can be scheduled. Caregiving means responding to whatever needs to be done now.

But there is an area in which you can and should set limits: the things you will do for yourself. For example, you will set aside time each day for the activities you enjoy. You will insist on going for a walk or to the gym or to a coffee shop by yourself. Whether you can leave your loved one alone for this time depends upon her condition. If it's necessary, have someone— a friend or a relative or a paid care aide—come in to sit with her while you're gone, even just to be there in case of an emergency. Remember, being an effective caregiver doesn't mean you no longer have your own life. You need some personal time. Insisting on it is a limit.

## Advice from Others

You will encounter well-meaning people anxious to offer you advice. They will suggest some treatment they heard about, or they will advise you to do things, like go on a vacation, that you just can't do. How do you handle this? Here's my policy.

If the advice comes from a health care professional, I'll listen and maybe even ask for a clarification. If it's from a layperson and I haven't asked for advice (and I usually haven't), I nod politely and instruct my short-term memory to translate whatever the person is saying into mumble-speak.

There is one type of advice I will listen to. If someone says something like, "I don't know if this will work for you, but I found it helpful," I'll pay attention. The person has acknowledged that the advice might not work and, more importantly, is speaking from experience instead of something he or she read in a supermarket checkout magazine.

One comment frustrates caregivers, including me. It's something like, "You're doing such a great job caring for your spouse." This is meant as a compliment, so why does it bother us? I believe there are two reasons. First, we caregivers seldom feel we deserve the kudos. We're so involved in providing care and we see so clearly the flaws and faults in what we're doing that the comment seems unearned. We feel we're struggling and stumbling so often that we're barely getting by and our daily battle is anything but great. I acknowledge the compliment, but my hidden sentiment is, *if you only knew*. Second, I have never met a caregiver who wants that role; becoming good at it is not one of our aspirations.

However, there is a comment that most caregivers I've met appreciate: "And how are you doing?" It demonstrates compassion.

# Hiring a Care Aide

For the past few years, almost everyone who knows about Sandra and her Parkinson's has advised me to hire a care aide. For that same length of time, I resisted. And I was wrong.

The advice was relentless. It came from friends and family, from doctors, from therapists—both physio- and occupational—from case managers, even from patrons of the coffee shop we frequent. And it was clear: hire a care aide. Why? Because you need a break; you need to look after yourself; you have to take time for you; you won't do Sandra any good if you collapse. So hire someone who can take some of the load off your back.

Now, I agree with all of these points; they're uncontroversial. So why did I reject them? Because I didn't need help. I was fine. Yes, caregiving was demanding and yes, it was frustrating. But I was handling it. So, no. Thank you, but I don't need help.

But Parkinson's is progressive and as Sandra worsened, so did the demands of giving care. One disheartening day, I reached the point where I finally had to acknowledge that I couldn't handle it adequately anymore. So I relented, hired a care aide, and prepared myself for the inevitable disruption that a stranger would bring and with it, perhaps a touch of relief.

And that's when I experienced one of the more humbling realizations of my life.

Within three days, Melissa, the care aide, was putting Sandra through range-of-motion exercises that I couldn't have done because I had neither the time nor the knowledge. She began to treat potential skin breakdowns from Sandra's time in bed: sores I'd seen but hadn't appreciated what they were. She spotted a couple of other emerging medical problems I would never have caught but that would have been serious had they developed. And she started what she called "pampering": giving personal care that I didn't know to provide. In other words, she was looking after Sandra better than I ever did or could have. And this shouldn't be surprising: she's a trained professional. I'm not.

Now my intent here is not to flagellate myself, but to point out how misguided everyone was who advised me to get help. By focusing on the benefits to me, they guaranteed I'd resist. I wish someone had shaken me and said something like, "Listen, bozo. It's not about you, it's about giving the best possible care to your wife." Sandra would have had the benefits several years earlier.

So my message to you caregivers who may be resisting hiring help is this: you do it for your loved one, not for you. Any relief you get is welcome, but it's a side effect because it's not about you, it's about the person who receives the care.

## Anger and Frustration

There will be times when you become angry or upset or frustrated and when your emotions lead you to say things that you later regret—which of course leads to guilt, which fuels your frustration, which . . . well, you get the picture.

Anger becomes even worse when you compare your reactions to those of good care aides or nurses who seem to have the patience of saints.

So how do you handle anger?

Above all, never let your anger slide into physical abuse. If you feel that starting to happen, get counseling. You're not helping your loved one or yourself, and you risk criminal charges. If you need to hit something, hit a wall or a door, or protect your hand and house by hitting a cushion. Or go into your backyard and scream. If the neighbors ask what's wrong, tell them you're practicing becoming a human bagpipe and invite them to your next recital. They'll leave you alone the next time you need to vent.

Second, don't compare your behavior to that of professionals. They also get angry, and they work in (usually) eight-hour shifts. You face the problems of caregiving all day, every day.

Finally, remind yourself that anger, confrontation, and reconciliation are parts of any sound relationship. Did you ever get angry at your loved one before he or she was diagnosed? I'll bet you did. So why should it be any different because your loved one needs care?

Don't confuse anger with frustration. I've asked Sandra if she'd like to go to the coffee shop or just have something to drink at home, and she hasn't answered me. I understand why and I'm not angry at her just because I have to repeat myself, but I am frustrated. That frustration leads me to speak louder (like the tourist who knows that the shopkeeper in some exotic location really does speak English if you yell loudly enough). That can seem like anger. It isn't. It's an attempt, which usually works, to get Sandra to state her preference.

At times she doesn't understand a simple question. I'll ask something like, "Do you want a piece of toast?" only to have her laugh. When I ask again, "Would you like some toast to eat?" she says oh and then answers me. What did she think I said? I have no idea, but at least it amused her—at the price of my frustration.

There's another reason I raise my voice. If Sandra is semi-asleep, I may say, loudly and sharply, "Wake up. Open your eyes." That's not anger. It's a strategy to get her to focus. Sandra called it a "pattern interrupt," a technique she used as a nurse. It doesn't always work, but it does so often enough for me to keep it as a tool.

After a bout of fury, I do a simple test: I ask myself if I've cooled down. If I have, then I know that what I felt was frustration. It was an episode, and there will be many more in my life. If I ever find I haven't calmed down—or worse, I don't want calm—then I will know that what I'm feeling is anger, it is becoming chronic, and I need to seek help.

I must confess, however, that I'm faster to anger than I used to be. Not toward Sandra, but toward the world. I'm less tolerant of others' errors, particularly those of strangers, than I once was. For example, one evening I was watching the news. One of the weather forecasters has an annoying habit of talking about "the overnight" or what was going to happen in "your overnight." I suddenly found myself furious, on my feet, and ready to throw something through the screen. I yelled, "Ditz! You can't say THE overnight. 'Overnight' isn't a noun." Grammatically, I was right, but my reaction was way out of proportion to the offense.

So I have to monitor my anger. So far, it hasn't prevented me from dealing kindly with friends or casual acquaintances, and I don't believe it has embittered me. If that day ever comes, I'll need to get therapy.

## The "Benefits"

At a meeting of our support group, a member asked whether caregiving had given us any benefits: something to be thankful for. I gave a glib answer, straight out of some heartwarming tract, about how it had made me stronger. But driving home, I realized that was nonsense: there were no benefits. If I felt anything, it was more like despair.

To be sure, there were some positives: anger is better than depression; I'd learned a great deal about Parkinson's and learning is always good; and

I'd met some great people in the support group. But there's a difference between positive effects and a positive situation. My situation, and that of everyone else in the group, was nowhere near positive. There was nothing to celebrate. There are no benefits.

But, you may object, many people claim to have benefited from some trauma because it made clear to them what's important in life. I don't doubt them. I recall a football player who lost a close relative, leading his coach to remind us that there are more important things in life than football. While I appreciated his sincerity and support for his player, I wondered who would ever have believed otherwise.

I doubt most of us really need teaching. Few would question the advice to leave work early to hug their kids. But few who receive that advice follow it. There are too many immediate distractions: that in-basket needs whittling down; that project needs attention; that report needs to be finished; I've earned some relaxation time with my buddies. I'll hug my kids tomorrow. I believe a traumatic event, far from teaching what's important, gives urgency: I'd better leave early today to hug my kids because I may not have the chance tomorrow.

Sandra's Parkinson's hasn't taught me anything about life I didn't already know. It's just focused me on dealing with it. And that's not a benefit, it's a duty.

## On Quitting

Someone once asked me a poignant question: if I had known in advance what was in store for Sandra and me, would I have remained with her or would I have left. Since I didn't know in advance, the question is hypothetical, and I never give, or trust, a categorical answer to a hypothetical question. For example, I once watched a panel discussion on a TV news channel about whether people who were HIV positive or had AIDS should be legally obliged to disclose their status to prospective partners. This is a complex question, but all of the panelists—whose qualifications to be on national television were not at all apparent—solemnly assured us that of course they personally would. My response was, "Bull." Nobody knows in advance how he or she will respond to a new situation. So the only answer I can give is that I hope I would have stayed with her.

I have met a few people who left when their spouses were diagnosed with a serious illness. At first, I was critical, but then I had a lengthy talk with a man who'd left his wife after she was told she had breast cancer. He was in distress about deserting her, but the diagnosis had made her bitter and angry, and she lashed out at the world, including him, even blaming him for her condition. He finally reached the point where he could no longer take the abuse.

Sandra has made it easy for me to stay with her. She has never lost her good cheer or her humor, and she always fights the disease, even when she has to spend most of her energy just surviving it. I overheard her on the phone saying of me, "He's always there for me. I'm really lucky." Lucky! I was choked up. And even on those days when she is almost unresponsive and I tell her I love her, she can still whisper, "I love you too."

So here's my advice. If you or a loved one receives a stark diagnosis, whether of Parkinson's or any other serious medical condition, talk it over. If you find that hard to do, get counseling. You are partners, committed to share one another's triumphs and support one another's problems. This is the time you need one another and you need to support one another. Yes, support goes in both directions: you need to support her, but she has to understand that she needs to support you. She needs to be there for you, if only by her attitude and her appreciation for all you do.

If you find that it's getting hard, that bitterness and anger are growing, seek professional help. As a partner, you are entitled to your loved one's support. As a caregiver, you need it. One writer prefers the term "care partner" to "caregiver."* I've stuck with the more traditional term in this book, but the distinction is particularly germane to this section.

## Living for Today

When motivational speakers aren't comparing people to frogs, one of their exhortations is "Live for today. Don't dwell on the past; don't live for the future." Beyond their entertainment value, I've never had much regard for motivational speakers, but having lived as a caregiver, I can say that this advice truly is bunk.

I'm a fulltime caregiver for Sandra. One of the distresses of that role is that living for today is all we have; we can't live for the future. We used to

---

\*    Christensen, page 128.

buy season tickets—an activity that is truly future-oriented—but we don't anymore because I can't predict that on an evening three months from now, or a week, or even tonight, she will be sufficiently "up" to go. So we can't plan. And if you're tempted to point out I still have to plan for what I'll do when I can no longer look after her, I'll just say you're confusing goal planning with contingency planning. Goal planning is getting ready for an extended vacation; contingency planning is buying travel insurance. Goal planning is getting ready to enjoy a long drive; contingency planning is making sure you have a spare tire and the tools to change it. In other words, goal planning is for something you look forward to, something you want to achieve. Contingency planning is preparing for an event you hope will never happen, or at least you won't welcome when it does.

If I can't plan or set goals, then my life boils down to eating, defecating, and sleeping, with the occasional episode of some forgettable television show to occupy my time. That's living for today. And it's full-time caregiving. Or it is unless you ignore the motivational speakers and live for the future to the extent you can.

How? With more modest goals.

Set a goal with your loved one that next Saturday, you'll get a wheelchair and hit the mall. Or on Sunday, you'll go for a long drive and maybe have coffee at that little place you found several years ago. Or on Wednesday, you'll rent or download that new Star Trek movie and make a batch of popcorn. That's next week. Not tonight, not spur of the moment, but next Wednesday. Make it a point that on one or two days in the week, you'll wake up with something to anticipate. And if on that day, your loved one can't handle the plan, well, change it. The point is not to carry it out (although most times, you will), it's just to have it. Plans provide something to look forward to.

Motivational speakers also denounce dwelling on the past. Since you can't change it, there's no point in focusing on it. Again, that's nonsense. Why? Because you need the past to remind you of the person your loved one used to be.

Today, Sandra is fully dependent on me. She needs me to help her get dressed, to feed her, to clean her. Because she has almost no ability to participate in her life, it's easy to fall into the trap of forgetting that wasn't always the case: to lose sight of the woman she once was.

Sandra was driven, attractive, fiercely loyal, infuriating, intelligent, biased, opinionated, stubborn, loving, caring, interfering, talented . . . Need I go on? You could make a similar list for your loved one. One of the great benefits of writing this book is that it forced me to dwell on the past. It confronted me with the memory of Sandra and made me appreciate how lucky I was to have met her and how much more complete my life became when she agreed to share hers with me.

And it isn't even right to speak of her attributes in the past tense. She still has them. They're muted, hidden beneath her struggles to make it through each day. But I can see glimpses of them, insights that make my life easier because when I look at her past, I know I'm not just dealing with a dependent burden, I'm dealing with a life partner. I'm not just acting out of duty, I'm also acting out of love.

So here's my other piece of advice. Every few days, take some quiet time and remind yourself who your loved one was. You don't need to write a book to remember her. Look at old photos. Pick a piece of her clothing and recall some funny thing that happened when she was wearing it. Play music that may have some meaning to you. And don't just focus on the good times. Remember the arguments, the tears, and the reconciliations. You can do this with her or by yourself. The point is to remind yourself of past times. But, you may object, isn't that depressing? Isn't that mourning what she's lost? It can be if you allow it, but that's not the point of the exercise. The point is to remind yourself why you've taken on the role of caregiver: out of the love and commitment that has enriched years of your life.

## And in Conclusion

I hope I've been able to give you some useful advice and tips on how to make your and your loved one's lives easier. There is far more available out there than I've been able to present. There are exercise therapies, massage, counseling, and a host of valuable services that may help you. The Internet is a rich trove of valuable information, and even if much of it is bogus, there are things that will help you and your loved one cope. Use these resources. Live well with them.

# 25

# The End of Caregiving

Sandra put up a valiant fight against her Parkinson's. But it's not a fight anyone ever wins. Sadly, in May 2017, after I had finished writing this book but before she could ever see it in print, she passed away. I decided to leave the rest of the book unchanged, as if Sandra were still here. Because in my heart, she is.

Just after New Year's, she came down with the flu and spent three weeks in hospital. For most of it, she was minimally responsive and on a nasal feeding tube. One of her doctors told me that if she didn't start swallowing, they would have to insert a feeding tube into her abdomen—and what kind of quality of life would that give her? That was a blunt, realistic question. The doctor's advice: start end-of-life planning. That was the toughest day I had faced.

A few times during our marriage, I had broached the subject of death with Sandra. Neither of us would live forever, and I wanted to know her preferences. But every time I raised it, she either ignored me or changed the topic. It was not something she was willing to discuss. So now, the decision was solely mine and I had to face the question: What will I do?

Then it struck me that if swallowing was the issue, she would damn well swallow. So the next day, I brought her a glass of water and a straw. By the end of the day, she had drunk half a glass, which delighted me and annoyed the nurse, who pointed out the posted order that she was to receive nothing by mouth.

She began to improve, and about a week later, after the doctor removed the feeding tube and she was eating solid foods, they discharged her.

But even though she was back home, she never recovered to where she had been before. The main symptom was that she stopped eating. Neither her care aide, Melissa, nor I could get food into her. I consulted with her doctor, who surmised that the disease had migrated to her brain stem and that she was near the end. He suggested she be put on palliative care.

Palliative care means keeping the patient comfortable without engaging in extreme medical interventions. Sandra was not in distress. She slept most of the time and had no pain, so there was little for the palliative care nurses to do but monitor her.

Yet even toward the end, she remained the feisty woman I loved. One evening, she refused to eat. On the advice of the palliative care team, I didn't try to push her, but I did ask if she wanted some ice cream. When she murmured yes, I got her a bowl, but when I tried to feed her, she clamped her mouth shut. I said, "This is ice cream. You like ice cream." No response. I complained, "But you asked for ice cream." In a clear, strong voice, she said, "I lied." I had to laugh. That was my Sandra.

Her sister Vivian arrived and was able to visit with her for a few days. Then on May 14, Mother's Day, her breathing became ragged and she was non-responsive. The palliative care nurse said she was near the end. Later that day when I checked up on her, she had passed away. She died comfortably, peacefully, in her own bed with me and her sister near her.

I arranged for her to be cremated. The following Saturday, I held a memorial for her. I conducted it myself. I've been to funerals where it was clear the person officiating hadn't known the deceased, and I wanted more for Sandra. At the memorial, I talked of her life, of her accomplishments, of her independence and strong will, and of my gratitude at having had her in my life.

After the memorial, family members came to the house. I had been concerned about her paintings. What would I do with them? I knew I'd be moving to a smaller place at some time and there wouldn't be room for them, but I hated the idea of abandoning them to strangers. So I invited family members to take any paintings they liked. I was gratified when people said how much they had always loved the one they selected, but watching them leave with their paintings—pieces of Sandra—was painful. I wanted to blurt out that I'd changed my mind. But even though it may have been too soon after her passing, it was the right thing to do. Her paintings are her legacy; every time someone looks at one, Sandra will be in their hearts.

The next day, with a few family members, I scattered her ashes at a spot we both loved. And I bid her good-bye.

There has not been enough time for me to recover, and we all grieve in our own way. But as a final postscript to this book, I'd like to pass on what I've been through in the hopes it may help those of you who, one day, will also face the end of caregiving.

People told me her death was the end of her suffering and of my struggles as a caregiver, and that, in a way, it was a blessing. I suppose that's true, but her passing was still sorrowful.

The reality is that I've been grieving her loss for several years. It wasn't a physical loss, but the woman I fell in love with was disappearing, and while I could see flashes of her spirit, they were more like shadows. The Sandra I was taking care of was not the Sandra I married. So even though her passing was a loss, it was the conclusion of an extended process.

People who had been through this gave me one priceless piece of advice: coast. I've allowed myself to shed all the "I should do this" prompts. In time, they will return—they are part of life. But for now, I'm allowing myself to wander. And I've learned a few truths.

I've learned that laughter is not disrespectful. I welcome it as a sign that I still have a life to live.

I've learned that I don't have to be stoic. When I look at something in a store and think, *Sandra would love that*, my eyes start to water. Kind, observant people have asked me if I'm all right. I thank them and reassure them that yes, I am. It's not quite true, but it's close enough.

I've learned how important family and good friends are. I've always appreciated them, but the relationships have shifted. In a way, they have become caregivers for me. Not in the physical sense, but in the support and concern they offer, and I love them for it.

And I'm beginning to evolve a new set of behaviors. Sandra and I used to watch television in the evening because it was the only thing we could do together. Now, I watch the news, but that's it. I rarely watch the programs we used to enjoy.

I find I'm eating better because I'm not too exhausted at the end of the day to make anything other than hot dogs or hamburgers or the occasional casserole.

Often, I find myself with time and nothing to do. That's a feeling I've never experienced before, and I still haven't figured out how to handle it, but I'm sure I will.

And finally, I am shaping a goal. I want to help caregivers deal with the pain and frustration that goes with the role. That was one motivation for this book. But now, it's become even more important.

Shortly after Sandra passed away, I saw a motto that brought tears to my eyes. I want to make it part of my life.

Live. Laugh. Love.

# Afterword

When I started writing this book, my motivations were unclear. It seemed important to me, but I wasn't sure why. And there was a powerful hesitation that caused me to consider not bothering.

Recalling the events, researching the disease, writing the book—all of this crystallized the book's value: it was therapeutic. But I still had a concern. I was worried about the effect the book might have on caregivers and on Parkinson's patients. I didn't want to be responsible for panicking my readers, causing them to flee from their loved ones. So I asked the members of my Parkinson's caregivers support group for their opinion. Every one of them said with enthusiasm, "Go for it."

So I did. If, after you read this book, you decide you can't face what's coming, let me state two things. First, you don't know what's coming. Sandra's journey is different from that of most other Parkinson's patients, just as theirs is different from one another's. Parkinson's has been called a "boutique" disease, but I prefer to think of it as a buffet. You don't know what symptoms your loved one will suffer, you don't know how severe they will be, you don't know how long they'll take to develop, and you have no idea what new treatments will become available.

Second, your decision to leave or stay won't come from anything you read. I can't influence anyone but me—and even that's shaky at times. I think those of you who decide to leave will leave anyway; it might just take longer. To those of you who decide to stay, I hope I've given you some insight into Parkinson's and some strategies for dealing with it.

Regardless of how you've been touched by this nasty disease and what you choose to do, I offer you my sympathy and my expectation that, however you deal with it, you will.

# Acknowledgements and Thanks

S andra didn't take her journey alone. Along the way, she had help, encouragement, and support from many people. I'd like to acknowledge and thank them.

To Sandra's family. To her sister Vivian Gordon, who, whenever she has opened her home to us, has always insisted we take the master bed because it's easier for Sandra. To her brother Gary Johnson and his wife, Helen, for having a sympathetic ear. To her sister Carol Beier and her husband, Pete, for their support.

To my family. To my brother, Nick Bloomfield, and his wife, Bev, for their many visits. Nick introduced Sandra to blonde jokes. She always scowled, but she always laughed at the same time. To my sister, Christine Reinke, and her husband, Glenn, for their support, their sympathy, and Christine's lively enthusiasm.

To our good friends. Many of the people we know drifted away after Sandra's diagnosis. You didn't. To Chuck and Trudy Lewis, whose "We'll bring dessert" is always welcome. To Bea Cunningham and to Alan King and Susan Izumi. Although you live at the other end of the country, when we get together it's always as if we just saw each other yesterday. To Della Bascom, Sandra's classmate and maid of honor, and to her gentle friend Ray Erskine.

To Sandra's doctors, who have helped her and demonstrated a great combination of compassion and capabilities. To our family doctor, Gidon Frame, and his associates and staff at the Old Orchard Medical Clinic. To Sandra's neurologist, Jeff Beckman, who had the unenviable task of giving her his diagnosis. To Larry Dian, with his welcome mix of empathy and knowledge. To Chris Honey, Sandra's neurosurgeon, and his remarkable skills and approachability. To Rodrigo Mercado and his deft touch at DBS programming. To Leslie Sheldon, whose program at St. Vincent's Hospital brought her back from a precipitous decline. To David Stuart, who guided her through her bout with DCIS with patience and understanding. To Andrew Howard, whose kindness, empathy, and skills boosted her performance when it seemed there were no other options available. To Silke Cresswell, her neurologist at the Pacific Parkinson's Research Centre, for her attempts to help Sandra cope.

To those who helped her with her DBS surgery. To Mini Sandhu and Nancy Polyhronopoulos, whose professionalism was a welcome addition to the DBS program. To Diana Herring, who found a combination of settings that gave her several years of function. And to the denizens of the DBS surgery Yahoo forum, who gave me more value than I can possibly repay.

To Quincy Almeida, whose Parkinson's rehabilitation program at Wilfrid Laurier University provided her with benefits that were visible years later.

To the professionals who helped her. To Shelagh Davies and her extraordinary talent in speech therapy. To Barb Taylor, her physiotherapist, who helped her recover fully from what could have been a devastating injury. To Melissa Daase, her care aide, who cared for Sandra both professionally and personally. To her case managers and the care aides at Burnaby Home Care. To the professionals at the Respite Hotel in Queen's Park Hospital. And to Manjit Deogan and the staff of Cranberry Cottage, Sandra's day program.

To the memory of our parents. To Betty and Sigfred Johnson, who gave Sandra to me. And to my parents, Murlis and Paul Bloomfield, who, I guess, gave me to Sandra.

To Frank Battista and his caring family, and to his friend Adora.

To Eileen Kernaghan, whose comments from her writing course have emboldened me to keep on putting pen to paper (or fingers to keyboard).

To Joyce Gram, my editor, who can always untwist my prose when it becomes entangled.

Finally, to the members of my Parkinson's caregiver support group, who have helped me more than I expected. To Deb, who holds us together, to Gisa and Jane and Eleonore and Richard and to the memory of Bergen. We're at different places on the journey, but we're all on it. And to Mike, who lost his wife to the disease. I enjoy the times we meet for coffee.

# APPENDIX A

# Sandra's Chronology

I have presented Sandra's journey more or less, but not entirely, chronologically. This is partly because sticking strictly to a time line would be confusing—so many things overlap—and partly because it made more sense to me to group topics together.

If I've done my job well, some of you may want to review one or two of the topics I've covered. So to help you, here is a chronology of her journey, along with the chapter where I've discussed it. I hope you find it useful.

| Date | Description | Chapter |
|------|-------------|---------|
| Oct. 3, 1996 | Sandra was diagnosed with Parkinson's. | 7 |
| Jan. 1, 2000 | She had surgery on her wrist to shorten her ulna. | 8 |
| Jan. 1, 2003 | We moved out of our office in downtown Vancouver. | 8 |
| Feb. 10, 2003 | She had a fine-needle biopsy that confirmed DCIS in her right breast. | 9 |
| Apr. 4, 2003 | She had her first consultation with the B.C. Cancer Agency. | 9 |
| Jun. 24, 2003 | She had a lumpectomy. | 9 |
| Sep. 3, 2003 | She started watchful waiting of the DCIS. | 9 |
| Sep. 30, 2003 | She had her first consultation on Deep Brain Stimulation (DBS) surgery. | 10 |
| Jan. 9, 2004 | She was admitted to St. Vincent's Hospital to have her medications adjusted. | 8 |

| Jan. 27, 2004 | A bone scan led to a diagnosis of osteoporosis. | 16 |
| Jun. 7, 2004 | She failed her driver's test. | 19 |
| Aug. 9, 2004 | She had DBS surgery. | 10 |
| Jan. 19, 2005 | Her driver's license was cancelled. | 19 |
| Feb. 22, 2006 | She started Lee Silverman Voice Therapy. | 11 |
| Nov. 23, 2006 | She fell and broke her acetabulum (hip). | 11 |
| Jan. 31, 2007 | She began to develop hallucinations, probably from the opioid medications. | 11 |
| May 1, 2007 | She consulted with a DBS programmer in Seattle. | 12 |
| Nov. 27, 2007 | She had her first urinary consultation. | 16 |
| Jul. 22, 2008 | She started Aclasta infusions. | 16 |
| Aug. 29, 2008 | She had the DBS electrodes removed and replaced. | 12 |
| Nov. 13, 2008 | She first entered respite. | 15 |
| Sep. 3, 2010 | She took the exercise rehabilitation program at Wilfrid Laurier University. | 18 |
| Jun. 11, 2011 | She had a sleep apnea study. | 16 |
| Jul. 14, 2011 | She consulted at the University of B.C. Pacific Parkinson's Research Centre. | 17 |

# APPENDIX B

# Parkinson's Medications

This is a list of medications used to treat Parkinson's and some of its symptoms. I have differentiated between the generic and brand name. The brand name is what a manufacturer calls a medication, while the generic name is what science calls it. For example, Aspirin is the brand name used by Bayer for acetylsalicylic acid (ASA), the generic name for the painkiller. Any pharmaceutical manufacturer can make ASA, but only Bayer can make Aspirin.

Before I present this list, I need to make two disclaimers.

First, the list is not complete. Even had it been at the time I wrote this, it wouldn't be shortly afterward.

Second, I have to be legalistic: THIS LIST OF MEDICATIONS IS INTENDED FOR INFORMATION ONLY. I take no responsibility for the effects of any of these medications on you or your loved ones. The medications you and your loved one take are up to the two of you and your doctors.

I've grouped the medications into four categories: "Levodopa medications," "Dopamine agonists," "Dopamine boosters," and "Other medications." For each medication, I've given the generic name, the brand names, and in a few cases a comment. Note that brand names may vary in different countries and that some medications may not be available where you are.

## Levodopa Medications

These medications are intended to increase the amount of dopamine by supplying levodopa, which will get converted to dopamine in the brain.

| Generic Name | Brand Name | Comments |
| --- | --- | --- |
| Levodopa/ carbidopa | Sinemet | Sometimes known as Sinemet IR, where "IR" means immediate release. |
| | Sinemet CR | "CR" means controlled release. |
| | Parcopa | |
| | Atamet | |
| | Duopa (U.S.) Duodopa (non-U.S.) | Given directly into the intestine by an external pump. |
| Levodopa/ carbidopa/ entacapone | Stalevo | Combines levodopa and carbidopa with entacapone (Comtan) to boost the effectiveness of levodopa. |
| Levodopa/ benserazide | Madopar | Benserazide is similar to carbidopa in that it prevents levodopa from being transformed into dopamine in the body. |

## Dopamine Agonists

Dopamine agonists are medications that mimic the effects of dopamine.

| Generic Name | Brand Name | Comments |
| --- | --- | --- |
| Pramipexole | Mirapex | |
| Ropinerole | Requip | |
| Apomorphine | Apokyn | Apomorphine medications are not given orally, but through injection or with a continuous pump. |
| | Ixense | |
| | Spontane | |
| | Uprima | |
| Bromocriptine | Parlodel | |
| | Cycloset | Cycloset is used primarily for type 2 diabetes. |
| Piribedil | Trivastal | |

| | | |
|---|---|---|
| Cabergoline | Dostinex | |
| | Cabaser | |
| Neupro | Rotigotine | Given with a skin patch. |
| Pergolide mesylate | Permax | No longer available in the U.S. |

## Dopamine Boosters

The term "dopamine booster" isn't a standard medical term. I use it here to describe medications that, in one way or another, increase the availability of the brain's existing levels of dopamine. For example, there is a chemical that breaks dopamine down, somewhat like a recycling depot. Some of these medications inhibit or block that chemical. By interfering with the breakdown of dopamine, it is expected that the smaller supply will last longer.

| Generic Name | Brand Name | Comments |
|---|---|---|
| Selegiline | Anipryl | |
| | L-deprenyl | |
| | Eldepryl | |
| | Emsam | Given as a patch. |
| | Zelapar | |
| Rasagiline | Azilect | |
| Benztropine | Cogentin | |
| Trihexyphenidyl | Artane | |
| Tolcapone | Tasmar | Was withdrawn because of liver damage; since re-introduced. |
| Entacapone | Comtan | |
| Amantadine | Symmetrel | |

## Other Medications

These medications are used to treat Parkinson's symptoms such as dementia or falling.

| Generic Name | Brand Name | Comments |
|---|---|---|
| Rivastigmine tartrate | Exelon | For treatment of Parkinson's dementia. Given as a patch or orally. |
| Clozapine | Clozaril | For treatment of Parkinson's dementia. |
| | FazaClo | |
| Modafinil | Alertec | For treatment of excessive daytime sleeping. |
| | Provigil | |
| Donepezil | Aricept | To help prevent falling. |

# APPENDIX C

# Glossary of Terms

| Term | Definition |
|---|---|
| Action tremor | A tremor that only occurs when the person is attempting some action. Also called an "intention tremor." |
| Activities of daily living (ADL) | A term used by occupational therapists. It refers to normal daily activities such as dressing, eating, or recreation. |
| Akinesia | An absence of movement. Freezing is an example. |
| Aspiration | The passing of food or fluids into the lungs instead of the stomach. |
| Biomarker | A physical characteristic, such as blood sugar levels, that indicates the presence of a medical condition. Currently, there are none for Parkinson's. |
| Blood-brain barrier | A filter that blocks some substances in the bloodstream from entering the brain. |
| Bradykinesia | Slowness of movement. Stiffness. |
| Bradyphrenia | Slowness of thinking and increased response time. |
| Carbidopa | A chemical that blocks levodopa from being converted to dopamine. It protects levodopa until it is delivered to the brain. |
| Cogwheeling | A ratcheting sensation in joints, particularly the wrist and elbow, in which movements are not smooth. This is a Parkinson's symptom. |
| DBS surgery | Deep brain stimulation surgery. It implants electrodes into a target in the brain and connects them to a pulse generator. It has been called a pacemaker for the brain. |

| Term | Definition |
|------|------------|
| Dementia | Cognitive problems, including memory loss, hallucinations, and loss of the ability to plan and manage one's life. |
| Dopamine | A neurotransmitter. Dopamine deficiency results in Parkinson's. |
| Dopaminergic | Refers to neurons that use dopamine as a neurotransmitter. |
| Dyskinesia | Uncontrolled writhing, twisting movements, usually of the head, arms, and shoulders. This is a medication side effect. |
| Dystonia | Painful, sustained muscle contractions. This can be a medication side effect, and it can also be a Parkinson's symptom or a separate condition. |
| Essential tremor | A medical condition characterized by a resting tremor. Essential tremor is sometimes confused with Parkinson's, but it does not carry the other parkinsonian symptoms. |
| Facial masking | A symptom of Parkinson's in which the patient's face loses expression. |
| Festination | Short, running steps that seem to accelerate. |
| Freezing | A form of akinesia or absence of movement while walking. The person who is freezing is unable to initiate walking without help. |
| Globus pallidus | An area within the brain that is one of two targets for DBS surgery. The other is the sub-thalamic nucleus. |
| Hypokinesia | An extreme slowness of movement. |
| Hypomimia | A lack of facial expression. Facial masking. |
| Hypophonia | Lowered voice volume. |
| Implantable pulse generator (IPG) | The battery pack and controls used to send electrical signals to the electrodes following deep brain stimulation surgery. |
| Intention tremor | A tremor that only occurs when the person is attempting some action. Also called an "action tremor." |
| Levodopa | A dopamine precursor. Levodopa is converted into dopamine. |

| Term | Definition |
|---|---|
| Lewy bodies and Lewy body dementia | Lewy bodies are clumps of protein in the brain that are associated with Parkinson's. They are also associated with some forms of dementia. |
| Micrographia | Small, cramped handwriting. |
| Neuron | A brain cell. There are about a hundred billion in a typical human brain. |
| Neuroprotection | A means to protect against the progress of Parkinson's. One focus of research is to find medications that are neuroprotective. |
| Neurotransmitter | A chemical that carries a neurological signal across a synapse: the gap between neurons. |
| Off-label prescription | A prescription of a medication for a purpose for which it hasn't been approved. Doctors may do this legally. |
| On-off fluctuations | The phenomenon in which a Parkinson's patient is benefiting from medications (on) or has lost the benefit prior to the next dose (off). |
| Pallidotomy | Surgery to destroy neurons in a region of the brain called the globus pallidus in order to control Parkinson's symptoms. |
| Parkinsonism | Any medical condition that has the same symptoms as Parkinson's disease, including Parkinson's itself. |
| Pill-rolling | A type of tremor in which the thumb and forefinger rub back and forth against each other. |
| Placebo | An apparent treatment that has no medical value. Used in research. |
| Placebo effect | An improvement in a medical condition as the result of taking a placebo. |
| Punding | An activity characterized by repetitive, mechanical actions. Resulting from dopamine overactivity, it is usually a side effect of medications. |
| Resting tremor | A tremor that occurs when the person is at rest. Contrasts with an action or intention tremor. |
| Scoliosis | An abnormal, side-to-side curvature of the spine. |
| Stereotactic frame | The frame used in deep brain stimulation surgery to guide the electrodes to their targets and to hold the patient's head steady. |

| Term | Definition |
| --- | --- |
| Substantia nigra | A region in the brain responsible for overseeing motor control and coordination. This area is impaired with Parkinson's. |
| Sub-thalamic nucleus | An area within the brain that is one of two targets for deep brain stimulation surgery. The other is the globus pallidus. |
| Synapse | The gap between neurons over which a neurotransmitter carries the neurological signal. |
| Thalamotomy | Surgery to destroy neurons in a region of the brain called the thalamus in order to control Parkinson's symptoms. |

# APPENDIX D

# Online Resources

In this section, I've listed the major national organizations in the United States in alphabetical order, followed by those in other countries. I've also included two for-profit organizations.

In addition to these, there are a vast number of local and regional organizations.

## Resources in the United States

**American Parkinson Disease Association** (www.apdaparkinson.org). "The American Parkinson Disease Association (APDA) was founded in 1961 with the dual purpose to Ease the Burden – Find the Cure for Parkinson's disease. As the country's largest Parkinson's grassroots organization, APDA aims to Ease the Burden for the more than one million Americans with Parkinson's disease and their families through a nationwide network of Chapters, Information and Referral (I&R) Centers, and support groups. APDA pursues its efforts to Find the Cure by funding Centers for Advanced Research and awarding grants to fund the most promising research toward discovering the cause(s) and finding the cure for Parkinson's disease."

**Lotsa Helping Hands** (http://lotsahelpinghands.com/) isn't specific to Parkinson's, but it "powers online caring Communities that help restore health and balance to caregivers' lives. Our service brings together caregivers and volunteers through online Communities that organize daily life during times of medical crisis or caregiver exhaustion in neighborhoods and communities worldwide. Caregivers benefit from the gifts of much needed help, emotional support, and peace of mind, while volunteers find meaning in giving back to those in need."

**The Michael J. Fox Foundation** (www.michaeljfox.org), an excellent source of information, was founded by the actor, who, like Sandra, lived in Burnaby. I hope it's not something in our air. "Fox Trial Finder" is a list of clinical trials seeking participants. One of its current programs is the Parkinson's Progressive Markers Initiative (PPMI), a study aimed at finding a biomarker for the disease.

**The National Parkinson Foundation** (www.parkinson.org) has partners in centers around the world. Its "Centers of Excellence" deal with Parkinson's research. NPF offers a range of publications and outreach programs. Merged with the Parkinson's Disease Foundation to form the Parkinson's Foundation.

**The Parkinson Alliance** (www.parkinsonalliance.org) is a national non-profit organization dedicated to raising funds to help finance the most promising research to find the cause and cure for Parkinson's disease. It also sponsors the Parkinson's Unity Walk and Team Parkinson. One of the organization's focuses is on patients who have undergone Deep Brain Stimulation surgery. Its website, www.dbs4pd.org, is a sound source of information about the procedure.

**The Parkinson's Disease Foundation** (www.pdf.org) is a national organization dedicated to funding research into the disease and acting as a source of information about it. One of the programs that PDF offers is the Parkinson's Advocates in Research (PAIR), a program that enlists people with Parkinson's and their caregivers to advocate for research and treatment programs. Their course is offered online. PDF also sponsors periodic webinars on various topics. Merged with the National Parkinson Foundation to form the Parkinson's Foundation.

**Parkinson's Foundation** (www.parkinson.org) is a merger between the National Parkinson Foundation and the Parkinson's Disease Foundation. It is carrying on the programs of both organizations.

**Parkinson's Resource Organization** (www.parkinsonsresource.org) is a 501(c)(3) non-profit charitable organization that provides group and individual support to those making the journey through Parkinson's. Funding for its programs comes primarily from donations by its members, donations to its monthly newsletters, and memorials.

**Medtronic** (http://www.medtronic.com/patients/parkinsons-disease/index.htm) is a for-profit organization that manufactures the stimulator most often used in DBS surgery.

**Medifocus** (www.medifocus.com). I've found their Guidebook on Parkinson's Disease to be valuable. There is a charge for the book.

## International Resources

These national organizations are similar to those in the United States in that they raise funds for research as well as support and education. Many of them, such as Parkinson Canada, have a number of provincial and regional societies. Some of these, particularly in smaller countries, are email addresses only. I have not tested them.

| | |
|---|---|
| Europe | **European Parkinson's Disease Association** (www.epda.eu.com/en/) is an umbrella organization that represents 45 national Parkinson's organizations in 36 countries. |
| International | **International Parkinson and Movement Disorder Society** (http://www.movementdisorders.org/) |
| Argentina | **Grupo de Autoayuda Parkinson Argentina** (http://aceparparkinson.wix.com/acepar) |
| Australia | **Parkinson's Australia** (http://www.parkinsons.org.au/) |
| Austria | **Parkinson Selbsthilfe Österreich** (www.parkinson-sh.at) |
| Belgium | **Association Parkinson francophone** (www.parkinsonasbl.be) |
| Brazil | **Associação Brasil Parkinson** (www.parkinson.org.br) |
| Bulgaria | **Fondazia Parkinsonism** (Email: wen.boss2@yahoo.com) |
| Canada | **Parkinson Canada** (www.parkinson.ca) |
| Chile | **Liga Chilena contra el Mal Parkinson** (www.parkinson.cl) |
| Croatia | **HUBPP – Hrvatska Udruga Bolesnika s Poremećajem Pokreta** (http://hubpp.mef.hr) |
| Cyprus | **Cyprus Parkinson's Disease Association** (www.cpda.org.cy) |

| | |
|---|---|
| Czech Rep. | **Spoleĉnost PARKINSON, o. s** (www.spolecnost-parkinson.cz or www.parkinson-brno.cz) |
| Denmark | **Parkinsonforeningen** (www.parkinson.dk) |
| Estonia | **Eesti Parkinsoniliit** (www.parkinson.ee) |
| Ethiopia | **Parkinson Patients Association – Ethiopia** (Email: parkinsonassociation11@gmail.com) |
| Faeroe Islands | **Parkinsonfelagið** (www.parkinson.fo) |
| Finland | **Suomen Parkinson-liitto ry** (www.parkinson.fi) |
| France | **Association France Parkinson** (www.franceparkinson.fr) |
| Georgia | **Georgian International Charitable Union of Parkinson's Disease Patients** (Email: pparkinsongeo@yahoo.com) |
| Germany | **Deutsche Parkinson Vereinigung e.V.** (www.parkinson-vereinigung.de) |
| Greece | **EPIKOUROS – Kinisis (Movement) Branch** (www.parkinsonportal.gr) |
| Hong Kong | **Hong Kong Parkinson's Disease Foundation** (http://www.hkpdf.org.hk/) |
| Hungary | **Delta Magyar Parkinson Egyesület** (www.fogomakezed.hu) |
| Iceland | **PSÍ – Parkinsonsamtökin á Íslandi** (www.psi.is) |
| India | **Parkinson's Disease and Movement Disorder Society** (www.parkinsonssocietyindia.com) |
| Ireland | **Parkinson's Association of Ireland** (www.parkinsons.ie) |
| Israel | **Israel Parkinson Association** (www.parkinson.org.il) |
| Italy | **Parkinson Italia** (www.parkinson-italia.it) |
| Japan | **Japan Parkinson Disease Association** (http://jpda-net.org/) |
| Korea | **Korean Movement Disorder Society** (http://www.kmds.or.kr/) |
| Lithuania | **Lietuvos Parkinsono ligos draugija** (www.parkinsonas.org) |
| Luxembourg | **Parkinson Luxembourg (PL) a.s.b.l** (www.parkinsonlux.lu) |
| Malaysia | **Malaysian Parkinson's Disease Association** (www.mpda.org.my) |
| Malta | **Malta Parkinson's Disease Association** (www.maltaparkinsons.com) |
| Mexico | **Asociación Mexicana de Parkinson A.C.** (http://www.ampac.org.mx/) |
| Netherlands | **Parkinson Vereniging (PV)** (www.parkinson-vereniging.nl) |

| | |
|---|---|
| New Zealand | **Parkinson's New Zealand** (www.parkinsons.org.nz) |
| Norway | **Norges Parkinsonforbund** (www.parkinson.no) |
| Pakistan | **Pakistan Parkinson's Society (PPS)** (www.parkinsons.org.pk) |
| Philippines | **Parkinsons Support Group of the Philippines Foundation Inc.** (Email: parkinsons.ph@gmail.com) |
| Poland | **Fundacja "Żyć z chorobą Parkinsona"** (www.parkinsonfundacja.pl or www.parkinson.net.pl) |
| Portugal | **Associação Portuguesa de Doentes de Parkinson** (www.parkinson.pt) |
| Romania | **Asociaţia Antiparkinson** (www.asociatia-antiparkinson.ro or www.parkinson.home.ro) |
| Russia | **The Regional Non-profit Organisation for the Advancement of Parkinsonian Patients** (Email: extrapyr@orc.ru) |
| Saudi Arabia | **King Faisal Specialist Hospital and Research Center Movement disorders program** (https://www.kfshrc.edu.sa/en/home/organization/493) |
| Serbia | **Serbian Association Against Parkinson's Disease** (Email: vladimir.s.kostic@gmail.com) |
| Singapore | **Parkinson's Society (Singapore)** (http://www.parkinson.org.sg/) |
| Slovenia | **Društvo TREPETLIKA** (www.trepetlika.si) |
| South Africa | **Parkinson's Disease & Related Movement Disorders Association of South Africa** (http://www.charitysa.co.za/parkinsons-and-related-movement-disorders-sa.html) |
| Spain | **Federación Española de Párkinson** (www.fedesparkinson.org) |
| Sweden | **ParkinsonFörbundet** (www.parkinsonforbundet.se) |
| Switzerland | **Parkinson Schweiz** (www.parkinson.ch) |
| Turkey | **Parkinson Hastalığı Derneği** (www.parkinsondernegi.com) |
| Ukraine | **Ukrainian Parkinson Disease Society** (www.geront.kiev.ua) |
| UK | **Parkinson's UK** (www.parkinsons.org.uk) |

# APPENDIX E

# Traveling Checklist

Going on a trip? Here's a checklist to help you make sure you have everything you'll need. Also, so you don't forget the things <u>you</u> need, the checklist has two columns: one for you and one for your loved one

| Item | My Loved One's | Mine |
|------|----------------|------|
| **Medications** | | |
| Parkinson's medications | ❑ | ❑ |
| Other medications | ❑ | ❑ |
| Nutritional supplements, vitamins, minerals, etc. | ❑ | ❑ |
| | ❑ | ❑ |
| | ❑ | ❑ |
| **Over-the-counter products** | | |
| Painkillers (Aspirin, Tylenol) | ❑ | ❑ |
| Motion sickness tablets | ❑ | ❑ |
| Diarrhea or constipation medications | ❑ | ❑ |
| Cough and cold medications | ❑ | ❑ |

| Item | My Loved One's | Mine |
|---|:---:|:---:|
|  | ❏ | ❏ |
|  | ❏ | ❏ |
| **Toiletries** | | |
| Special soaps | ❏ | ❏ |
| Creams, lotions | ❏ | ❏ |
| Aftershave | ❏ | ❏ |
| Deodorant | ❏ | ❏ |
| Toothpaste | ❏ | ❏ |
| Toothbrushes | ❏ | ❏ |
| Cosmetics and makeup | ❏ | ❏ |
|  | ❏ | ❏ |
|  | ❏ | ❏ |
|  | ❏ | ❏ |
| **Prosthetics** | | |
| False teeth | ❏ | ❏ |
| Eyeglasses | ❏ | ❏ |
| Contact lenses | ❏ | ❏ |
| Contact lens cases and cleaners | ❏ | ❏ |
| Hearing aids | ❏ | ❏ |
| Batteries | ❏ | ❏ |
|  | ❏ | ❏ |
|  | ❏ | ❏ |

| Item | My Loved One's | Mine |
|------|:---:|:---:|
| | | |
| | ❏ | ❏ |
| | ❏ | ❏ |
| **Mobility Devices** | | |
| Cane | ❏ | ❏ |
| Walker | ❏ | ❏ |
| Wheelchair | ❏ | ❏ |
| Portable bed rail | ❏ | ❏ |
| | ❏ | ❏ |
| | ❏ | ❏ |
| | ❏ | ❏ |
| **Personal Hygiene** | | |
| Adult diapers | ❏ | ❏ |
| Wet wipes | ❏ | ❏ |
| Rubber gloves | ❏ | ❏ |
| Facial tissue | ❏ | ❏ |
| Bed pads | ❏ | ❏ |
| Bottled water | ❏ | ❏ |
| | ❏ | ❏ |
| | ❏ | ❏ |

| Item | My Loved One's | Mine |
|---|:---:|:---:|
| **Documentation** | | |
| Contact information for family members | ❏ | ❏ |
| Family doctor's contact information | ❏ | ❏ |
| Health insurance documentation | ❏ | ❏ |
| Passports, visas | ❏ | ❏ |
| Special instructions for medical staff | ❏ | ❏ |
| List of allergies | ❏ | ❏ |
| Medications and doses and times they're given | ❏ | ❏ |
| | ❏ | ❏ |
| | ❏ | ❏ |
| | ❏ | ❏ |
| | ❏ | ❏ |
| **Others** | | |
| | ❏ | ❏ |
| | ❏ | ❏ |
| | ❏ | ❏ |
| | ❏ | ❏ |
| | ❏ | ❏ |
| | ❏ | ❏ |

# APPENDIX F

# Questions Regarding DBS

I f you or your loved one is considering deep brain stimulation surgery, here is a list of questions for your neurosurgeon. Some of these are the ones Sandra and I had for Dr. Honey, although I've modified the list because some of ours no longer apply. For many of these, I've given answers in italics. Where there is no answer, it will vary from one surgeon to another. Some of the answers reflect what I believe is current knowledge, although you should verify this with your neurosurgeon who is, after all, the expert.

## General Questions about DBS

1. When do you recommend having DBS surgery?

   *Neurosurgeons no longer regard DBS surgery as a treatment of last resort or as experimental. It has become a standard treatment option based on the patient's condition and readiness.*

2. Does DBS surgery protect against the progress of the disease?

   *There is no evidence of this.*

3. What's the impact on speech?

   *There is evidence that DBS surgery worsens speech in some patients.*

4. How does DBS surgery affect dyskinesia?

   *Dyskinesias result from too much medication. Because DBS surgery reduces the need for medication, it's possible that the combination of medications and stimulation results in a condition similar to overmedication. If this happens, the stimulus needs to be modified and the level of medications adjusted.*

5. How about dystonia?

   *As with dyskinesia, preventing dystonia requires adjusting the stimulus and the medications.*

6. What symptoms is DBS surgery most useful for?

   *The same ones that levodopa medications treat, particularly tremor, and to some degree stiffness.*

7. How about depression or dementia?

   *There's no evidence that DBS surgery worsens cognitive functions.*

8. There are two targets: sub-thalamic nucleus or globus pallidus. Which is best?

   *This is the neurosurgeon's preference. There doesn't appear to be any clear evidence one way or the other.*

9. For how long is DBS surgery effective?

   *This is still being tracked. Most analyses suggest that it is effective for five years, but there are numerous cases of people benefiting ten or even twenty years later, including Sandra, who has had DBS implants for over twelve years.*

10. Is anything else coming along that would lead you personally to defer surgery?

## Hospital and Surgical History Questions

11. What are your hemorrhage rates?

    *Ideally, 1% or less.*

12. What are your infection rates?

    *Ideally, 2% or less.*

13. What precautions do you recommend to prevent post-operative infections?

*[We didn't ask this question because Sandra was a nurse. But the answer is to keep the area clean and above all dry. Getting it wet is an invitation to infections.]*

14. The more procedures a surgeon has performed, the lower the rate of complications. How many of these procedures have you and this hospital performed?

    *Over 100 is good.*

15. There have been reports of problems following electrode placement, usually cognitive and speech issues, which may be related to damage to the sub-thalamic nucleus (STN) during electrode placement. Is the STN damaged during surgery?

    *Ideally not, but sometimes damage is unavoidable.*

16. Is there lesioning of the brain when the electrodes are placed, and if so, what are the effects?

    *There can be slight lesioning. Typically, there are no effects.*

17. Different sites have different procedures. Please describe what you do here in terms of

    - Number of procedures
    - The duration of each
    - The time between them
    - Hospital stays
    - Recovery times

    *During Sandra's surgery, there was just one procedure, but some hospitals have up to three: one for each electrode and one for implanting the stimulator. Sandra's surgery lasted nine hours and she stayed in hospital for one day afterward.*

18. Do I take my Parkinson's medications prior to surgery?

    *No.*

19. Are there nutritional or herbal supplements that I should avoid prior to or after surgery?

    *Gingko biloba, ASA (Aspirin), blood thinners.*

20. How are patients weaned off their existing medications?

    *That's done during programming.*

21. Other than pre-operative antibiotics, what medications do you administer before, during, and after the surgery?

22. Those who have undergone DBS report that the qualifications, availability, and helpfulness of the programmer are critical. Who does the programming and what are his or her qualifications?

    *Ideally, a separate full-time programmer, usually a nurse trained in DBS programming.*

23. What is the availability and waiting list for DBS programming or adjustments?

    *Sooner is more desirable.*

24. Is there a pool of programmers so if one is on vacation, another is available, or if one is not satisfactory, another can be called?

    *Ideally, yes.*

25. Does the programmer provide a copy of the printout after each programming session?

    *Ideally, yes.*

26. How much of the head is shaved?

## Effectiveness of the Procedure

27. What is the incidence of cognitive, speech, or other problems, and are these problems solvable with therapy, programming, or removal of the DBS device?

    *There may be tradeoffs. For example, relief of tremor versus diminished speech. That's a decision for the patient.*

28. Does having the DBS implants restrict vigorous activities?

    *It shouldn't.*

29. Is there a risk that ongoing activities can disrupt the placement of the components?

    *Not usually.*

30. Is there a risk that scar tissue will build up around the leads and restrict head and neck movements?

    *Some people report that they can feel the leads pulling.*

31. After the surgery, will I be able to drive? Work? Dance? Hike? Golf?

*Probably, assuming you could before.*

## Ongoing Maintenance

32. Other than the surgical procedure itself, is there any ongoing discomfort with the placing of the components in the chest?

*No.*

33. What are the day-to-day requirements for tending to the system? That is, once it is set, can I leave it alone, or do I have to make ongoing adjustments to it?

*You may be able to make adjustments as you need to, but those are for your convenience. Any other maintenance will be done by the DBS programmer or the neurosurgeon.*

34. Is there a need to adjust the system to accommodate for external factors such as stress?

*Not unless you find it helps.*

35. Is there a capability to make adjustments myself?

*The programmer may provide a range of settings, such as voltage levels, within which you can make adjustments.*

36. Are there ways to test that the system is intact and working properly, such as testing the quality of the signals?

*This is part of programming.*

37. Does the presence of the electrodes interfere with or militate against future diagnostic functions such as CT or MRI?

*You can have CT scans or diagnostic ultrasound without concern. Not MRIs. Absolutely do not have one without the approval of a neurosurgeon trained in DBS surgery. Also do not have any form of diathermy, including ultrasound diathermy.*

38. When the battery dies, is there any advance warning, and if so, how much?

*The remote controller gives battery levels and warnings. When you get a low battery signal, contact the DBS clinic immediately.*

39. How complex is the replacement procedure?

    *Day surgery.*

40. How quickly can you do it?

41. What precautions do I need to take with respect to magnetic devices such as security systems in stores or airports?

    *You will receive a card exempting you from airport security. Security systems in stores aren't usually a problem.*

42. How about proximity to computer monitors, telephone headsets, speakers, etc.?

    *Not a problem.*

43. Can the system be removed should that be called for?

    *Yes.*

44. Do you recommend a Medic Alert bracelet, and is there a standard wording that medical staff will recognize?

    *That's up to you.*

# Bibliography

Bandler, Richard. (1993). *Time for a Change*. Capitola, CA: Meta Publications.

Birtwhistle, J. and D. Baldwin. "Role of dopamine in schizophrenia and Parkinson's disease." *British Journal of Nursing* (1998): vol. 7, no 14: 832–41.

Bordelon, Yvette M., et al. "Medication responsiveness of motor symptoms in a population-based study of Parkinson disease." (2011). Retrieved from http://www.hindawi.com/journals/pd/2011/967839/.

Braak, Heiko, et al. "Staging of brain pathology related to sporadic Parkinson's disease." *Neurobiology of Aging* (2003): vol. 24, no 2: 197–211.

Boyles, Salynn. "Parkinson's: later diagnosis, earlier death." (2010, October 4). Retrieved from http://www.webmd.com/parkinsons-disease/news/20101004/parkinsons-later-diagnosis-earlier-death.

Breast Cancer. DCIS—"Ductal Carcinoma In Situ." (2013, September 9). Retrieved from http://www.breastcancer.org/symptoms/types/dcis.

Bronstein, Jeff M., et al. "Deep brain stimulation for Parkinson disease." *Archives of Neurology* (2011): vol. 68, no. 2: 165.

Burke, Robert E., William T. Dauer, and Jean Paul G. Vonsattel. "A critical evaluation of the Braak staging scheme for Parkinson's disease." *Annals of Neurology* (2008): vol. 64, no. 5: 485–491.

C-Health. "Parkinson's disease (shaking palsy)." (n.d.). Retrieved from http://chealth.canoe.com/condition/getcondition/parkinsons-disease#Symptoms.

_____. "Drug factsheets. Sinemet." (n.d.). Retrieved from http://chealth.canoe.com/drug/getdrug/sinemet#AdverseEffects.

Cheng, Hsiao-Chun, et al. "Clinical Progression in Parkinson's Disease and the Neurobiology of Axons." *Annals of Neurology* (2010): vol. 67, no. 6: 715-725.

Cherry, Kendra. "Identifying a neurotransmitter." (2017, July 5). Retrieved from http://psychology.about.com/od/nindex/g/neurotransmitter.htm.

Christensen, Jackie Hunt. (2005). *The First Year—Parkinson's Disease*. New York: Penguin Group.

Clarke, Carl E. (2001). *Parkinson's Disease in Practice*. London: Royal Society of Medicine Press.

Cram, David L., Steven H. Schechter, and Xiao-Ke Gao. (2009). *Understanding Parkinson's Disease*. 2nd ed. Omaha: Addicus Books.

Davis, Charles Patrick and Melissa Conrad Stöppler. "Parkinson disease dementia (cont.)." (n.d.). Retrieved from http://www.emedicinehealth. com/parkinson_disease_dementia/page3_em.htm.

Fink, J. Stephen. "The placebo effect in clinical trials in Parkinson's disease." (n.d.). Retrieved from https://www.apdaparkinson.org/the-placebo-effect-in-clinical-trials-in-parkinsons-disease/.

Fox, Michael J. (2003). *Lucky Man*. New York: Hyperion.

_____. (2009). *Always Looking Up*. New York: Hyperion.

Graboys. (2008). *Life in the Balance*. New York: Union Square Press.

Goldman, David A. and David A. Horowitz. (2000). *Parkinson's Disease*. New York: Dorling Kindersley.

Greene, Paul E. and Stanley Fahn. "Status of fetal tissue transplantation for the treatment of advanced Parkinson disease." *Neurosurgical Focus* (2002): vol. 13, no. 5: 1–4.

Grimes, David A. (2004). *Parkinson's Stepping Forward*. Toronto: Key Porter Books.

Hariz, Marwan I., Patric Blomstedt, and Ludvic Zrinco. "Deep brain stimulation between 1947 and 1987: the untold story." *Neurosurgical Focus* (2010): vol. 29, no. 2: E1.

Heyn, Sietske N. and Melissa Conrad Stöppler. "Parkinson's disease (cont'd)." (2013, December 4). Retrieved from https://www.medicinenet. com/parkinsons_disease/article.htm#what_is_the_prognosis_of_ parkinsons_disease.

Honey, Christopher D. and Manish Ranjan. "Deep brain stimulation for Parkinson's disease—a review." *US Neurology* (2012): vol. 8, no. 1: 12–19.

Iwasaki, S., et al. "Cause of death among patients with Parkinson's disease: a rare mortality due to cerebral haemorrhage." *Journal of Neurology* (1990): vol. 237, no. 2: 77–79.

James, Oliver. (2008). *Contented Dementia*. London: Vermilion.

Jha, Shivkumar and Walter A. Brown. "Depression in Parkinson disease." *Psychiatric Times*. (2006, November 1). Retrieved from http://www. psychiatrictimes.com/articles/depression-parkinson-disease.

Kieburtz, K., et al. "Effect of creatine monohydrate on clinical progression in patients with Parkinson disease: a randomized clinical trial." *Journal of the American Medical Association* (2015): vol. 313, no. 6: 584–93.

Laurier. "Welcome to MDRC." (n.d.). Retrieved from https://www.wlu.ca/homepage.php?grp_id=2234.

Levy, Robyn Michelle. (2011). *Most of Me*. Vancouver: Greystone Books.

Michael J. Fox Foundation. "Parkinson's Disease Prognosis." (n.d.). Retrieved from https://www.michaeljfox.org/understanding-parkinsons/living-with-pd/topic.php?prognosis&navid=prognosis.

Milo et al. *Nucleic Acids Research* (2010): vol. 38, no. 1: D750–D753.

Montague, Read. (2007). *How We Make Decisions*. New York: Penguin Group.

Montgomery, David. "Rush Limbaugh on the offensive against ad with Michael J. Fox." *The Washington Post*. (2006, October 25). Retrieved from http://www.washingtonpost.com/wp-dyn/content/article/2006/10/24/AR2006102400691.html.

Mosley, Anthony D. and Deborah S. Romaine. (2004). *The Encyclopedia of Parkinson's Disease*. New York: Amaranth.

National Institute of Neurological Disorders and Stroke. "Statement on the termination of QE3 Study." (2011, June 2). Retrieved from http://www.parkinson.org/understanding-parkinsons/what-is-parkinsons.

National Parkinson Foundation. "What is Parkinson's disease?" (n.d.). Retrieved from http://www.parkinson.org/understanding-parkinsons/what-is-parkinsons.

Parashos, Sotirios A., Rose Wickmann, and Todd Melby. (2013). *Navigating Life with Parkinson Disease*. New York: Oxford University Press.

Parkinson, Dr. James. (1817). *An Essay on the Shaking Palsy*. London: Sherwood, Neely, and Jones.

PHRMA. "Medicines in development for Parkinson's disease." (n.d.). Retrieved from http://www.phrma.org/report/medicines-in-development-for-parkinson-s-disease-2014-report.

Ross, G.W. and H. Petrovitch. "Current evidence for neuroprotective effects of nicotine and caffeine against Parkinson's disease." *Drugs & Aging* (2001): vol. 18, no. 11: 797–806.

Schrag, A., Y. Ben-Shlomo, and N. Quinn. "How valid is the clinical diagnosis of Parkinson's disease in the community?" *Journal of Neurology, Neurosurgery, and Psychiatry* (2002): vol. 73, no. 5: 529–534.

Schwarz, Shelley Peterman. (2002). *Parkinson's Disease: 300 Tips for Making Life Easier*. New York: Demos Medical Publishing.

Sharma, Nutan and Elaine Richman. (2005). *Parkinson's Disease and the Family*. Cambridge, MA: Harvard University Press.

Stem Cell Network. "Parkinson's disease." (May 2012). Retrieved from http://www.stemcellnetwork.ca/index.php?page=parkinson-s-disease&.

Tagliati, Michele, Gary N. Guten, and Jo Horne. (2007). *Parkinson's Disease for Dummies*. Hoboken, NJ: Wiley Publishing Inc.

Tapias, Victor, Jason R. Cannon, and J. Timothy Greenamyre. "Pomegranate juice exacerbates oxidative stress and nigrostriatal degeneration in Parkinson's disease." *Neurobiology of Aging* (2014): vol. 35, no. 4: 1162–1176.

Tuchman, Margaret. (n.d.). "Welcome." Retrieved from http://www.dbs4pd.org/.

University of California, San Francisco. "Gene therapy for Parkinson's disease." (n.d.). Retrieved from http://pdcenter.neurology.ucsf.edu/professionals-guide/gene-therapy-pd.

Veazey, Connie, et al. "Prevalence and treatment of depression in Parkinson's disease." *The Journal of Neuropsychiatry and Clinical Neurosciences* (2005): vol. 17, no. 3: 310–323.

Watkins, P. "COMT inhibitors and liver toxicity." *Neurology* (2000): vol. 55, no. 11, Supplement 4: S51–56.

WebMD. "Nerve pain and nerve damage." (n.d.). Retrieved from https://www.webmd.com/brain/nerve-pain-and-nerve-damage-symptoms-and-causes#1.

_____. "What is the placebo effect?" (n.d.). Retrieved from http://www.webmd.com/pain-management/what-is-the-placebo-effect.

Weiner, William J., Lisa M. Schulman, and Anthony E. Lang. (2007). *Parkinson's Disease*. 2nd ed. Baltimore: Johns Hopkins University Press.

# Index

not quitting, 177–8
notifications for emergency
  services, 145–7
office closure, 67–8
on caregiving "benefits," 176–7

relationship with Sandra, 168–9,
  170–1, 177–8
relationships with others, 169
on Sandra's death, 183–4
self-care, 158, 171–2
travel in Europe, 41–3
wheelchair ramp, 81, 150–2
Hallows, Sandra
  and airport wheelchairs, 88–9
  alternative medicine therapy,
    58–60
  anxiety, 134, 135
  appointments and tests, 103–5,
    124–5
  artist, 50, 182–3
  breast cancer scare, 71–3
  chronology, 188–9
  clinical trial, 62–5
  cognitive decline, 90–3, 133
  dating and marriage, 15–17,
    21–3, 29–31
  day program, 98
  death, 181
  decision-making, 20, 133
  deep brain stimulation (DBS)
    surgery, 38–40, 74–8, 84–6
  diagnosis announcement, 9, 58
  diagnosis date, 50, 58
  driver's license, 109
  education and career, 21–3, 29,
    48, 87–8
  on escalators, 107–8
  exercise rehabilitation program,
    106–8
  falls and injuries, 124–5, 132–3,
    159
  family, 27, 36–7

family misdiagnosis, 27
first name (Doris), 96
hallucinations, 82–3, 85–6, 134,
  135–6
hip fracture physiotherapy, 81–2
hospital reunion trip, 110
hypnosis therapy, 48–9, 67
infertility, 43–4
legal representation, 160
medications, 66, 68, 85–6, 103,
  145, 147–9, 163, 164
memorial, 182
non-recognition of Jolyon, 92
office closure, 67–8
osteoporosis, 99–100
osteotomy, 67
outings, 149
palliative care, 182
passport application, 35–6
personality, 21–3, 87–9, 180, 182
private care aide, 174–5
rating scale scores, 107
relationship with Jolyon, 168–9,
  170–1, 178
relationships with others, 169
respite care, 96–7, 157–8, 172
restrooms, 152
sleep apnea study, 101–2
speech therapy, 79–80, 133
symptoms, 60–1, 68
travel and end of, 109–13
travel and work in England, 41–2
travel in Europe, 41–3
urinary consultation, 100–1
vision decline, 102
weight loss and in-patient
  program, 68–70
wheelchair, 150–2
hallucinations, 52, 53, 82–3, 85,
  134–6
Herring, Diana, 84–5
hip fractures, 81–2
Hoehn and Yahr scale, 26

Holy Cross Hospital, 30, 97

home access, emergency services, 144–5

home assessments, 137–8

home care programs, 94–6

home preparation
  adaptations around the house, 143
  assistive devices, 138–40
  bedrooms, 141–2
  beds, 141, 142
  commodes, 141
  doors, 141
  flooring, 138
  home assessments, 137–8
  for incontinence, 142
  showers, 139–40
  staircases, 141
  toilets, 138–9, 141–2
  towel racks, 140

homeopathy, 69

Honey, Dr. Chris, 39, 74–5, 85, 86, 166

hotels, 111, 153–4

Howard, Dr. Andrew, 104–5, 135, 136

hypnosis therapy, 48–9, 67

**I**

implantable pulse generator (IPG), 76–8, 84–6

incontinence, 142

instability, 25

insurance (medical), 160–1

intention tremor. *See* tremor

**J**

Johnson, Betty (mother of Sandra Hallows), 37

Johnson, Esther (sister of Sandra Hallows), 27

Johnson, Sigfred (father of Sandra Hallows), 37

**L**

Lee Silverman Voice Therapy (LSVT), 79–81

legal issues (defense and representation), 158–60

levodopa medication, 32–3, 34, 38, 64–5, 130, 191

licensed nurses (LPNs), 122

Limbaugh, Rush, 33

lock boxes (home access), 144–5

**M**

mastectomy, 71–3

meal time, 128–9

medical alert systems, 143–5

medical insurance coverage, 160–1

medical professions, 121–2, 161–3

medical research
  clinical trials, 61–5
  exercise programs, 106–8

medical supply stores, 129, 130, 137–9, 142, 149, 150

medication administration policy, 156

medications
  administration, 129–30, 147–9
  blister packs, 147, 148–9, 165
  charts, 148
  daytime sleepiness, 193
  dementia, 193
  deterioration of, 149
  evaluations of, 163–4
  falls prevention, 193
  lists, 190–3
  "off-label use," 101, 164
  opioid, 82–3
  pillboxes, 148, 149
  pumps, 130, 191